THE PLACE OF
PHYSICAL EDUCATION IN SCHOOLS

Kogan Page Books for Teachers series
Series Editor: Tom Marjoram

THE PLACE OF PHYSICAL EDUCATION IN SCHOOLS

Edited by

——Len Almond——

Books for Teachers

Series Editor: Tom Marjoram

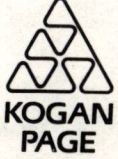

KOGAN PAGE

First published in 1989 by
Kogan Page Ltd
120 Pentonville Rd, London N1 9JN

British Library Cataloguing in Publication Data
The Place of physical education in schools
  1. Great Britain. Schools. Curriculum subjects
  Physical education
  I. Almond, Len
  613.7'07'1041

  ISBN 1-85091-692-6

Typeset by BookEns, Saffron Walden, Essex
Printed and bound in Great Britain by
Biddles Ltd, Guildford

Contents

List of Contributors

Len Almond:
Senior Lecturer in the Department of Physical Education and Sports Science, Loughborough University and Director of the HEA Health and Physical Education Project.

David Bunker:
Lecturer in the Department of Physical Education and Sports Science, Loughborough University.

Bernard Dickenson:
Physical Education Advisor, Sandwell.

Colin Hardy:
Lecturer in the Department of Physical Education and Sports Science, Loughborough University.

Jo Harris:
Lecturer in the Department of Physical Education, College of St Paul and St Mary, Cheltenham.

Bob Smith:
Lecturer in the Department of Physical Education and Sports Science, Loughborough University.

Bryan Smith:
Outdoor Education Teacher, Coventry.

Rod Thorpe:
Senior Lecturer in the Department of Physical Education and Sports Science, Loughborough University.

Introduction

The 14–18 curriculum has seen the advent of TVEI, CPVE, the new GCSE, and soon Records of Achievement will become a major feature of all teaching. These innovations have involved many teachers of physical education and they have required the learning of new skills in planning courses for accreditation and involvement in more and more meetings as consultation across different departments has become a necessity. The review of the school curriculum initiated by many local authorities has added to the work-load of teachers and involved them in a questioning of their role in school. The new Education Act and its implications for the work of schools and liaison with parents and other interested parties has created additional work for teachers and inevitably further stress.

In addition, teachers of physical education have had to experience a realignment of their responsibilities as directed time has made a big impact on the traditional practice of extra-curricular commitments after school and at week-ends. During 1987 they had to cut back drastically on school sport commitments and fend off the criticisms of some governing bodies of sport who accused teachers of not doing their job properly. This experience made many teachers re-examine how they use their time in extra-curricular commitments and has led to a crisis of conscience for teachers who have worried about their talented pupils and the opportunities for further development. This debate about school sport and the resulting inquiry into its problems has led many local education authorities and governing bodies of sport to re-examine the provision for the development of individual talent and the future development of their sport for the young, and to instigate new structures for the promotion of sport. These new structures and rethinking processes that many sporting bodies are engaged in have significant implications for the physical education curriculum.

The questioning of roles in the school curriculum, the changing status and position of school sport and the requirement of

9

heads of physical education departments to engage in school policy making have contributed to the feeling that there is a lack of a clear direction for physical education. Teachers have been conscious also of an absence of support structure to enable them to justify physical education and produce a coherent rationale that would stand up to the questioning of different departments. The skills of defending one's arguments, writing policy statements and matching aspirations with day-to-day practices go far beyond the traditional strengths of physical education teachers who are used to the practical world of sport.

In this context there is an urgent need to provide teachers with a framework for a curriculum that incorporates traditional interests and is disciplined by aspirations which can be justified on educational grounds. Thus, this need for an educational rationale for physical education which is clearly linked to a curriculum framework that will guide practice is a priority that teachers are desperately crying out for. This is not to say that physical education teachers are merely followers and are unable to produce their own rationale. The reality of the current teaching situation and the varying demands on both teachers' time and energy effectively creates an environment in which the construction of a coherent statement outlining the value of physical education for young people and its translation into practical exemplars is an almost impossible task for teachers. What is needed is a statement that will provide common ground for teachers to debate and to reflect upon in order that their own thinking can be informed by the constructive reactions of their colleagues.

In such a debate, critical reflection on a common document with colleagues will provide the base from which teachers can learn to discuss, to listen and to learn something of the way physical education impinges on the lives of those who teach it in schools. In this way common ground (rather than a consensus) among teachers will have the chance to emerge and this will inform the evolution of a teacher-based statement about the values of physical education.

It was this notion and the many requests from teachers for a coherent statement on the value of physical education in schools that led me to put together a book for teachers of physical education covering the age range 8–16. The reasoning behind my justification for physical education in the school curriculum is not that of a philosopher or a sociologist, but a curriculum developer who believes that it is important for teachers to reconstruct their own understandings of the value of physical education. I am merely providing the starting point for debate and inviting criticism from the whole profession so that teachers can benefit from the ensuing discussion, but at the same time I recognise that teachers need to have something to fall back on as an interim measure. This is important in the current climate.

In planning the contributions of different authors I drew upon those colleagues who have worked with me over a number of years. However, I had two further reasons behind my selection. During the past five years physical education has been involved in a number of major innovations which have been presented to teachers because they challenge traditional practices and provide a change of focus. It is important that these innovations contribute to the debate about the place of physical education in schools because they raise a number of significant issues and they represent the problematic nature of physical education. Because of their problematic nature, they provide the means by which key issues can be brought into the debate and they can contribute to the development of our understanding about the values of physical education. However, this understanding needs to be considered in the context of change that is rapidly overtaking all teachers and provides the backcloth in which any deliberation about the values of physical education must take place. Hence, I have included contributions from colleagues who are critical observers of the process of change in physical education. Such contributions provide us with cautionary tales and make us careful of jumping on to bandwagons that lead us up blind alleys or dead-ends.

I have divided this book into three parts. The first part provides a framework for the physical education curriculum supported by educational arguments which discipline the selection of appropriate activities and provide a structure to inform the practices of teachers. This is followed in Part 2 by a number of chapters outlining innovations that propose a change of focus for traditional activities. In Part 3 innovations that cross all of the activity-based foundations of physical education are introduced because they have already started to make an impact on the physical education curriculum and they will influence any debate about the future direction of our teaching.

Jerome Bruner spoke about the 'unfinished' curriculum when

he discussed the innovation of *MAN: A Course of Study* (a humanities curriculum for the middle years of schooling) on an in-service course with teachers who were preparing to introduce this innovative programme into the curriculum of their schools. In this sense this book represents the same image as Jerome Bruner's 'unfinished' curriculum because it is meant to stimulate debate and provide a starting point for teachers' own reconstruction of the values of physical education in the curriculum of all schools.

References

Bruner, J (1970) *MAN: A Course of Studies* Education Development Centre, Cambridge, MASS.

Part 1

Chapter 1
The Place of Physical Education in the Curriculum

Len Almond

Introduction

In this chapter I shall propose three significant reasons why physical education has a role to play in the school curriculum. This will be followed by an outline of how these proposals can be translated into practical possibilities to structure the selection of purposeful physical activities.

Why physical education should be included in the curriculum

Physical education contains a number of activities like sports, dance, and adventure activities which are human practices of great significance that affect people in a very pervasive manner and have become a fundamental part of human heritage and culture. Such activities take up a great deal of media space in newspapers, occupy many hours of radio and television, and throughout the world millions of people find them an absorbing interest and devote a lot of time to participation in them. At certain times international festivals of sporting excellence, for example the Olympic Games, World Championships for athletics, World Cup for soccer, arouse a great deal of interest, and are the source for much political and social debate. They have inspired people in the art world like musicians, artists, poets, writers and film producers to create works that have contributed to a deeper understanding of these cultural forms. Adventure in the outdoors, the natural environment and the wilderness represent both a source for satisfying curiosity and a challenge for the expression of human endeavour. Dance and performing arts are a constant source of inspiration and delight to both spectator and performer. Thus, within the field of human endeavour, sports, dance, and adventure pursuits represent an important and significant aspect of cultural life.

It has been argued that one of the tasks of schools is to promote access to, and engagement in, cultural forms and practices in order that young people can come to understand and recognise their significance (Lawton, 1975; Skilbeck, 1984). Thus, the curriculum becomes the means by which children can encounter and become acquainted with important and significant aspects of cultural life. This means that young people can learn to participate in sports, dance, and adventure activities which contain practices and rich traditions that exemplify human endeavour and are regarded as being valuable and worthwhile. Hence, it is important to recognise and acknowledge their significance within a culture because any form of educational enterprise concerned with such traditions would be incomplete without their inclusion.

There is a certain risk in describing the curriculum in terms of an initiation into a cultural tradition, because there is a tendency to represent tradition as something fixed and unchallengeable. Thus, cultural initiation becomes the transmission of the status quo, a commodity handed down from generation to generation, which is far from satisfactory if cultural forms and practices are defined exclusively in narrow terms and contain only the interests of dominant groups.

There is a need to go beyond the simple transmission of cultural forms and examine the transformative power of understanding derived from studying and engagement in sports, dance, or adventure activities. It is important to recognise that over time some traditional activities lose their appeal as interests change, and as developments occur in technology they provide the means for new sports to arise, and also provide scope for the opening up of new adventure/wilderness challenges. Schools need to recognise their role in stimulating new interests and widening perspectives about the richness and potential of the vast range of pursuits possible. Coming to understand this scope and recognising its significance and impact within our culture and tradition is an important aspect of school life.

Following from this argument that initiation into cultural forms and traditions should involve a study of sport, dance and adventure activities, it is important to recognise their contribution to the enhancement of an individual's quality of life. Such pursuits have been invented by people because they have the power to enrich life, become an absorbing interest which rewards and fulfils, provide avenues for the pursuit of human excellence and the development of human capacities and qualities, and enable people to explore their own potentialities.

Physical education in schools provides the means by which people can learn how to participate and become involved in sporting activities, dance and adventure activities (ie purposeful physical activities) so that they are able to make choices and select activities which can contribute to the enrichment of their lives and enhance the quality of their lives. At this point, it is important to recognise that purposeful physical activities represent only one curriculum source for enriching the quality of people's lives. Even though physical education in schools has the capacity to transform and enrich lives, it is important that pupils go beyond this so that their engagement, appreciation and subsequent reflections contribute to an understanding of their world and illuminate their perspective within this world. As a consequence, this engagement, appreciation and reflection will enable them to make informed decisions about what to do with their lives, and how they choose to spend their time. For some people (after engagement in various ways of spending their time and subsequent reflection), this may involve a rejection of sporting activities and the decision to choose, for example, music instead because for them it provides more scope for developing an absorbing interest and enrichment. For others it may involve a deeper commitment to a particular physical activity for the same reasons. It is important that in a school's provision for engagement in activities (including purposeful physical activity) which can enrich lives, the process of deliberation and reflection should be included in order that pupils can make sense of their situation and illuminate their understanding of what to do with their lives and how they choose to spend their time. One aspect of the 'practical' that Warnock (1988) argues for so elegantly.

Purposeful physical activity can be important both in and for people's lives by enhancing well-being. By promoting the enhancement of the body through engagement in physical activity it is the person who benefits not simply the body. The body's organs and systems need activity in order to develop them. Unlike a machine they do not wear out with appropriate use, but are strengthened by activity and impaired by lack of use. This inbuilt necessity for activity in order to promote the appropriate use of the body's organs and systems is an important feature of our human nature. As a consequence of being strengthened by activity a state of enhanced functioning provides energy to enrich life and generates feelings of well-being which promote the 'good' of a person, enabling human nature to flourish, a point developed by Von Wright (1963) in his analysis of the varieties of goodness.

A state of enhanced functioning is important, because adequate functioning is a relative term and differs according to people's circumstances. Thus, patients lying in bed unable to use their legs will accommodate to this condition by adjusting (in an integrative sense) the functioning of various systems to an appropriate but adequate state which meets all existing needs. In the same way, a sedentary person will accommodate to a routine of inactivity and adjust their functioning capabilities to meet appropriate needs. These adaptations with their integrative function create a homeostasis which ensures that people are unaware of their reduced functioning capabilities until they have to react to something like climbing a long flight of stairs or suddenly running to catch a bus. In this state 'feeling good', as a result of enhanced functioning brought about by a more active life-style that incorporates regular aerobic exercise, is unlikely to occur. In these states the 'good' of the individual or person is not being promoted, because human nature is unable to flourish.

In understanding oneself as a physical organism and how one's well-being can be promoted, a person would need to learn a great deal of practical knowledge concerning the growing body and its needs, the relationship of exercise with the health and welfare of an individual and how it can be protected and enhanced; a person would need to know how to exercise safely and correctly, how to make decisions about the role of physical activity within a life-style and how it can be incorporated into the routine patterns of daily life. Here, it is not simply a matter of acquiring knowledge about human behaviour, but coming to understand something of the complex inter-relationships of a person as a living whole, and acting on this understanding to promote the 'good' of a person. In making sense of such understanding, engagement in purposeful physical activity and the acquisition of a practical knowledge base about the enhancement of a person's well-being can play an important part in the education of young people.

So far, I have attempted to identify three specific areas in which physical education can make a contribution to the education of young people in schools. These areas are outlined as follows:

1. An initiation into purposeful physical activity so that individuals can understand and recognise their significance as important features of our culture. In addition to transmitting such cultural practices, it is necessary to examine their transformative power in developing a richer appreciation of culture and contributing to its development.
2. The deliberation and articulation about the role of purposeful physical activity in enhancing the quality of life in order to illuminate people's understanding of what to do with their lives and how they choose to spend their time. Such understanding requires the engagement in purposeful physical activities so that a person is able to make an informed choice.
3. Purposeful physical activity can be important for people's lives, because it is part of our understanding about the promotion of a person's welfare and well-being.

Thus, the education of young people would be incomplete if physical education was neglected and not recognised for the unique contribution that it makes through its concern with purposeful physical activity, to 'understanding', 'personal autonomy', and the development of 'persons'.[1] It may be that teachers in schools may wish to use physical education in other ways which are more instrumental than my outline. Physical education can be seen as some form of emotional catharsis, a release of pent up energy or relief from the boredom of academic study (a point recognised by many pupils when interviewed about why they do physical education (Dickenson, 1987)). It could also be used as some kind of socialising process or as a way of promoting the communal life of a school. Exercise could be seen as a means of making young people fitter, or simply as therapy for those pupils with some form of psychological dysfunction. In the same way, physical education could be used, in a narrow sense, to teach young people about the problems of cardiac risk factors and how exercise can play some part in the alleviation of such diseases. However, these instrumental reasons are insufficient on their own to justify physical education within a school curriculum, even though for some people they may add to the value of physical education.

As soon as the physical education teacher has identified reasons for the inclusion of the subject into the school curriculum which are acceptable to the profession and to educational colleagues, they need to be translated into practical possibilities which discipline the selection of appropriate activities and the nature of this content. It is here that I believe many problems occur within the physical education profession because we do not know what consensus exists about our purposes for the subject, and consequently there appears to be much disagreement as people debate the role of competitive sport, fitness, recreational activities, or the place of dance for boys, and mixed classes of boys and girls for physical education.

In some cases, this apparent disagreement arises from the lack of opportunity for debating such issues and talking them through adequately at different levels. However, after listening to much of this debate with teachers, I believe the nature of the disagreement between opposing views is not because teachers have different values, but it is due to the different weights (White, 1982) that teachers apportion to similar activities. Also, the gap between translating purposes into practical possibilities is too wide, therefore there is little apparent relationship between the two. As a consequence, it is not surprising that there is disagreement when there are few principles to discipline and guide the selection of activities.

In this chapter I intend to move beyond a statement of purposes, to outline a framework which serves to discipline and guide the selection of activities within a physical education curriculum. First, it is important to recognise that physical education in schools covers the age range 4–18, therefore it is crucial to appreciate the specific contributions of physical education within this wide range. In order to do this I propose that this wide range be seen in terms of three phases:

- Phase one: early years 4–7;
- Phase two: middle years 8–13; and
- Phase three: upper secondary 14–18.

Within these three distinct phases, it is necessary to acknowledge that there will be a need to highlight a specific emphasis on certain aspects of physical education. However, a concern for continuity and development must be shown in the planning of a curriculum for all three phases. Therefore, it is important for teachers to recognise within a specific phase where physical education is going and where it has come from. Each phase cannot be seen in isolation.

Phase one: the early years 4–7

The focus during this phase should emphasise the Management of the Body in Action acquired in the context of:

- expressive movement forms; and
- games.

I do not intend to develop this phase in detail because this book is for teachers working in the middle years of schooling and above. However, it is important to indicate some key aspects of Phase one in order to make connection between the phases.

Management of the body in action is a major feature of this phase, therefore it is necessary to formulate the following framework to illustrate its scope:

1. Biological functioning components:

- organs and systems of the body
- musculo-skeletal body.

2. Competence in basic fundamental movement patterns:

- locomotor/manipulative/stability

in

- different environments.

Young people take delight in the opportunity to be active and become involved in attempting/trying physical challenges. In schools we need to use this motivation and provide opportunities for young people to widen their experience of physical challenges in a range of different environments, for example water, gymnasia, and on playing fields, because they provide a rich potential of possibilities: to use the body expressively; to explore and experiment with different movement patterns; to learn how to practise in order to improve and progress; and to learn new ways of play through games. Learning to manage, co-ordinate, and control their bodies in purposeful physical activity, acquiring a range of motor competencies, and extending their physical capacities are important because they contribute to the development of a growing person.

In this way physical education can provide a foundation base from which the development of more disciplined forms of purposeful physical activity can emerge, and from which the promotion of physical well-being can be extended. However, it is important that teachers ensure that young people in the early years experience as wide a range of physical challenges as possible, and have the opportunity of learning to control and have mastery over their movement.

During this phase it may be necessary to make provision for work from the early years to continue beyond the age of seven because, for many reasons, it has been impossible to cover adequately the main features of this phase. In some schools teachers may be able to consider introducing features of Phase two at an earlier stage because they have more specialist help, more time devoted to physical education, or simply that their pupils are ready and able to undertake more advanced work. The critical point to recognise is that schools, teachers, and pupils can have different needs, therefore the teacher's professional judgement is important when it comes to deciding that sufficient sampling of the potential of physical education has been accomplished and pupils are ready to encounter new challenges.

Phase two: the middle years 8–13

The focus during this phase would be on three distinct aspects. The first one is concerned with what I call 'disciplined forms of physical activity' which are distinctive features of purposeful physical activity, with their own unique form that provides their significance and determines the satisfactions aroused by participation. They have evolved from 'management of the body in action' which forms the roots for the development of disciplined forms of physical activity. These forms fall into three categories:

1. Sports which provide an opportunity for the mutual quest for excellence in competitive situations with others.

2. Dance which provides an opportunity for the expression of aesthetic and artistic experiences and the capacity for stimulating imagination, sensitivity, and the appreciation of movement.
3. Adventure activities which provide challenges for the expression of human endeavour in the outdoors, the natural environment and the wilderness.

They are disciplined because they require dedication, striving to acquire complex skills and movement patterns, and thorough preparation for competitions, festivals, performances before an audience, and expeditions.

The second aspect is health and well-being which is concerned with:

- facilitating healthy growth and development;
- arousing feelings of well-being as a result of engagement in physical activity; and
- stimulating feeling good about oneself.

This aspect is a continuation of one major feature of 'management of the body in action' from Phase one, the promotion of biological functioning components to enhance the 'good' of a person.

The third aspect is difficult to define in precise terms therefore for want of a better term I shall call it an 'alternative activity curriculum'. This is a contrast to the disciplined forms of physical activity because it is important to provide pupils with the opportunity of learning about purposeful physical activity where the tensions of preparation and the need to acquire difficult competencies are more relaxed. Some people find satisfaction in engagement in physical activity of different sorts because they provide the opportunity for solitude, or calmness as well as the stimulation of movement. For some people physical activity can simply be a play activity which provides both a recreation, relaxation, and an opportunity for an absorbing interest with no pressure.

I have included Eastern Movement Form within this aspect because it is a genuine alternative to competitive sport and activities like Tai Chi provide opportunities for movement with lack of tension, balanced relaxed posture, an emphasis on slow respiration, and slow, smooth actions. As such they are purposeful physical activities with the capacity for people to learn about their potentialities, their physical limitations, to acquire knowledge about control of their bodies, and an awareness of the inner self. Such activities take place in a relaxed atmosphere and do not involve any form of ranking of pupils, social comparisons of performance, or grading. These forms of movement deserve our attention as potential sources for enhancing our understanding of physical education, and for providing opportunities for people to engage in purposeful physical activity. They enhance our understanding of the richness and potential of physical education, because they challenge us to think in different ways about the kind of values associated with purposeful movement. They also represent an important aspect of the transformative character of cultural practices, because they contribute to and enlarge our understanding.

I made the point earlier that in order to develop a curriculum for physical education, it is necessary to go beyond a statement of purposes and translate them into practical possibilities which discipline the selection of curriculum content. I now propose to select two aspects from Phase two and identify principles to guide teachers' selection of content. As sport, which is just one aspect of disciplined physical activity, represents a major feature of contemporary physical education, it provides a good opportunity to restate the value of such activities and to demonstrate how its important features can be highlighted. A health focus within physical education has become a major innovation in recent years, therefore this provides a good opportunity to clarify its central features.

SPORT EDUCATION

The current physical education curriculum is dominated by sporting activities but they appear as separate blocks or units within a programme and there is little attempt to establish relationships between these separate activities and teach young people about sport. Pupils simply experience a variety of different sports in isolation. Thus, in the first year of secondary education boys of 11 are likely to encounter soccer, rugby, cricket, athletics, cross-country running, swimming, and gymnastics. Girls would encounter netball, hockey and rounders to replace so-called boys' games. In some schools boys and girls may be taught in mixed groups, but the idea of girls and boys learning different games would still exist. Following this pattern in the second, third and fourth years the major changes would be the introduction of a wider range of games and less time spent on major team games like soccer, hockey, netball, and rugby. One of the main features of this pattern is the dominance of small units or blocks of work, often about six weeks, when pupils change activities. Consequently, there is little opportunity for an emphasis on continuity, development, and linking what is learnt in different years.

In order to change this state of affairs, I would like to propose that teachers consider the idea of *sport education* instead of teaching a wide variety of discreet sporting activities. The task for teachers is two-fold:

1. Initiate young people into a range of sporting activities which illustrate their significance as important aspects of cultural life.
2. Demonstrate how engagement in sporting activities can enrich people's lives and improve its quality so that they are able to illuminate their understanding of what to do with their lives and how to spend their time.

Thus, it is important that teachers go beyond simply providing the opportunity to engage in a variety of sports. Instead, they should sample and select activities which are representations of distinctive types of sport because of the vast range of sporting possibilities; there is also a need to teach much more than just engagement in physical activity. One such classification (Alderson, 1982) provides us with a useful way of making such a selection. He suggests the following sport activity types which are based on distinctive forms of ability and represent distinct aspects of motor control:

- coincidence anticipation – games;
- pattern replication – gymnastics; and
- power production – athletics (sustained or explosive).

As there is an enormous range of sporting possibilities with only limited resources in terms of facilities, staffing, finance, and time, it is necessary to use such a classification as a basis for allocating different kinds of sports to a particular category of sport type and making a selection for inclusion in the curriculum in order to achieve balance.

Once teachers have made their selection what features should they emphasise in addition to mastery of techniques and skills which are fundamental to sporting achievement? The following features are important aspects of learning about sport and an engagement in its traditions and practices.

The role of festivals

One of the attractions of sport within cultural traditions is a festival or a bringing together of competitors to share in the satisfactions aroused by participating in that sport, or to provide the opportunity for people to challenge worthy opponents. The culminating nature of a festival provides a base for teachers to use as a 'representation' of major events, but also as a means of bringing together everything that needs to be learnt for sport education.

Sport involves different roles

Within a festival, there are performers, coaches who support them and have been involved in the preparation for the events, and officials who oversee the conduct of the competitions. Thus, it is important that young people recognise that sport requires people who will adopt different roles and who serve different functions in the promotion of sport. Schools can provide the means by which young people have the opportunity to experience different roles in order to recognise their significance, but also to learn the different satisfactions that can be gained from participation as an official or a coach. In addition, it would be appropriate to provide opportunities for learning to be an informed spectator.

In schools, young people engage in sport usually as a performer and this is right, but there comes a time when it is necessary to provide the opportunity for them to act as a coach or leader of a small group preparing for a tournament, and also learn how to be an official. When young people are in their final two years of secondary education, some may decide that acting as a sports official is what they would choose to do as a leisure pursuit rather than be a performer. It is therefore important that we consider how we can make provision for such interests (or stimulate such interests). Obviously this will create many difficulties in terms of organising the acquisition of knowledge and experience for such roles and this must not be underestimated, but if we value the need to teach young people about the richness and potential of sport this is necessary. For many young people this aspect will take place much later in Phase two, while for others it will have to wait and become part of Phase three.

Learning to compete
This is a major aspect of sport education because competition is a necessary condition for sport. However, there is much confusion and misunderstanding about its use. I therefore propose to expand this section in order to articulate a view of competition which I believe provides much scope for considering what has to be learnt in an education which involves competitive sport.

Prior to the competitive experience of taking part in a competition, I believe it is necessary for young people to have had the opportunity to experience challenges where they have recognised that they are the agents of their own personal improvement, and where success is not based on comparison with others, for example rank order in a race. Athletics is usually presented in a form where pupils race against each other over, eg, 70 metres in order to provide a rank order of performance and produce a personal time, which reinforces, every time they race, that individuals who are less mature, or whose body-clock runs more slowly, are going to be ranked low. These pupils know they are going to be way behind their more mature peers and they have little incentive to improve or recognise progress if social comparison is the means for reinforcing behaviour.

Instead it may be more appropriate to ask individuals to run for four seconds (on different occasions it may be seven or ten seconds) and record with the help of a partner how far they have run. This can be repeated and the pupil can assess their achievement. When this is repeated three times, pupils usually exceed or they are very close to their previous performance. Thus, by switching the focus of achievement pupils are able to recognise improvement but also strive to extend their own performance. When pupils have gone through this kind of striving to improve their own achievements, they may wish to compare themselves with others, and they may choose to opt into competition. A sports education provides the opportunity for pupils to enter into formal competition against others.

At this point, a further distinction needs to be made between what I call competition in a weak sense and also a strong sense. If I choose to play badminton against another person, my motive is to have a good run around and enjoy the game. My opponent may be playing to test his skills. Both players need a rule structure in order for the game to proceed whereby each player will strive to score points and eventually someone will be acknowledged as the winner. In this situation winning is subservient to having a good game and satisfying each other's motive for playing the game. Even though competition is a necessary condition for the game it does not follow that winning is the sole point of engaging in this game of badminton; a point so vividly portrayed by Arnold (1979) in his description of two competitors in a game.

In the same way, young people will play games where the score is kept but it is not of lasting importance. This is competition in a weak sense. On the other hand, if the university decides to organise a squash tournament for staff I may enter because I want to win and move up the ladder. In this sense I am speaking of competition in a strong sense.

When young people play games the rule structure is merely the means to enable an activity to get underway, whereby points (or goals) are won or lost, and by which an opportunity is provided for satisfying individual motives; they are competing but are not in a competition in a strong sense. To take part in a formal competition is more complex and young people should not be forced into it. It should be something they wish to opt for because of the satisfaction associated with it. Some people will not be ready for the competitive experience and may not wish to enter into it. We need to respect this right.

Competition is a mutual quest in which rules exist to provide a structure for playing, but also for the 'good' of all participants who should be required to respect each other as worthy opponents. Thus, in the context of schools, teachers can endeavour to foster morally acceptable attitudes which discipline one's actions in competitive situations. This involves promoting a morality of aspiration (Miller, 1988) which is far more demanding than a morality of duty in which participants merely comply with the rules or stick to the letter of the law. Promoting a morality of aspiration or morally acceptable attitudes requires that teachers recognise and acknowledge the following:

1. The need to teach young people to play to win fairly (Meakin, 1986).
2. Opponents are not obstacles to one's success, it is the problems they present that represent the obstacle.
3. Victory or winning, if it is to be significant, requires outplaying worthy opponents not eliminating them.

4. Winners are not good, or losers bad and inferior, which appears to be accepted in conventional morality.
5. If participants in a competition wilfully violate the rules they are intentionally violating 'the good of all' because they are failing to adhere to the rules which they have agreed to by entering into a rule-defined contest.
6. The final score in a competition is only part of the picture because the impact of the experience of competing has wider implications.
7. Encourage competitors to value playing and competing more than simply winning.

Thus, the teacher who promotes competitive sport is engaged also in the nurturing of ideals which goes beyond conventional morality or even mere compliance with rules. The nurturing of ideals is concerned with promoting morally acceptable attitudes which discipline action, in other words a morality of aspiration. This will require treating competitors as ethical persons and considering very carefully the environment in which competition is promoted. Thus, the teacher or coach responsible for a team is of special importance because their words and actions, or what they expect of competitors as ethical individuals, create a climate or ethos which can support morally accepted attitudes or reinforce negative competitive values. Teachers and coaches of school teams need to display integrity, trust and respect, and provide role models that support a morality of aspiration and foster such attitudes in pupils. Finally, it may be necessary to create practical dilemmas in competitive situations that emphasise ethical positions so that morally acceptable attitudes can be reinforced.

In promoting morally acceptable attitudes and developing the idea of sport education, teachers could provide opportunities for young people to discuss and reflect on contemporary sports practices that they see in live situations, on television, or read about in newspapers. Such opportunities may be appropriate for humanities, English, or social science courses, but sport education would be impoverished if schools did not attempt to incorporate discussion and critical debate about such issues.

I have attempted to outline some critical aspects of learning to compete because they are important for the development of sport education. This is a powerful challenge to all teachers of physical education because this is a crucial issue of ethical importance and as educators we must respond to it positively.

Preparation for competition
Taking part in a festival or culminating event requires thorough preparation if one is to enhance one's performance and compete to the best of one's capabilities. Thus, it is necessary to plan and organise one's preparation with definite goals in mind and to strive to accomplish them. Such preparation will involve practising and refining techniques and skills, discussing with peers your strategies and tactics, and planning your training sessions to ensure that your physical conditioning is adequate. It will be necessary to consider the organisation of the culminating event or mini-festival which may be a first year tournament in basketball, a tutor group badminton competition, or a class cross-country competition. It is important to involve the pupils in such enterprises because they provide the opportunity for important learning experiences.

A HEALTH FOCUS IN PHYSICAL EDUCATION
The role of exercise and regular physical activity in the promotion of health has been identified and firmly established (Powell and Paffenbarger, 1985), but how can this be translated into a clear focus for teachers of physical education and what does this focus involve?

A concern for health within physical education should be associated with promoting:

- active lifestyles; and
- safe and correct exercise.

Active lifestyles
Here the teacher needs to plan activities in such a way that pupils are:

- stimulated to seek further participation in physical activity;
- able to learn how to gain satisfaction from participation and regard it as a good experience;
- able to enhance their self-esteem in the context of exercise; and
- able to recognise that everyone can be good at exercise.

The argument presented here is that if pupils' experience of physical activity and exercise within the normal physical education programme is one which they find satisfying and generates good feelings, rather than some kind of aversion therapy where exercise is a negative experience, it is likely that they will wish to repeat these experiences. Young people need to feel that they are capable of taking part in physical activity, whether it is a sporting activity or dance, and have the confidence to participate fully. Many pupils don't participate because they have been led to believe that they must learn the skills first. This strong over-emphasis on skill development may well be counter-productive in promoting active life-styles. We need to look carefully at our approach to stimulating and promoting further participation beyond the school.

In the same way, we need to teach young people that progress and improvement come from the belief that they are capable of achievement, and that everyone can feel good about their performance. Many people associate exercise with elite performers and not themselves. We need to convince all pupils that everyone can be good at exercising which means being aware of what all our pupils do, recognising their progress and acknowledging it as success.

Safe and correct exercise
The promotion of active life-styles needs to be supported by the intelligent performance of safe and correct exercise so that pupils have the opportunity of gaining knowledge and understanding of how to exercise, what kind of exercise is appropriate, and how to perform exercise safely and correctly. This kind of knowledge and understanding is relevant to courses on fitness for sport as well as courses which emphasise the health benefits of exercise.

However, safe and correct exercise for active life-styles needs to be underpinned by the idea of a practical knowledge base. Such a knowledge base needs to be acquired and experienced in a practical context rather than viewed as some kind of theoretical study which is classroom based. This is a further illustration of Warnock's notion of a practical curriculum (Warnock, 1988). This is important because a health focus in physical education which is concerned with knowledge can be construed as a classroom activity, and not seen as practical and applied knowledge acquired through action for action, where pupils can demonstrate that they 'know and understand'. Thus, it is important that teachers recognise the need for acquiring a practical knowledge base in the form of experiential learning in a practical context.

Such a knowledge base should involve the following aspects:

1. Exercising safely and correctly.
2. Cardiovascular health:
    - nutritional balance and the role of exercise in maintaining a stable body weight; and
    - stamina/endurance exercise for health benefits.
3. The role of exercise in developing a sound musculo-skeletal structure (including bone mineralisation).
4. The relationship between physical activity and the alleviation of stress.
5. Learning how to incorporate exercise into one's life-style.

Such a focus will require examining the traditional activities of physical education to identify their scope for teaching safe and correct exercise, so that the practical knowledge base is acquired as a deliberate emphasis rather than a mere spin-off, also it will require the introduction of new modules to teach those aspects that cannot be covered in athletics, swimming, gymnastics, games or dance. In the same way that GCSE, TVE, and CPVE have created a new look to the 14–16 curriculum it will be necessary to create new courses or modules which will have to replace some sport-based units. However, teachers will need to examine the role of health education in their school and consider whether some of this work can be incorporated successfully within it.

Phase three: upper secondary 14–18

The focus during this phase should be concerned with *life-style enhancement* so that students (no longer referred to as pupils) can intelligently choose from a variety of cultural forms those activities which can contribute to promoting the quality of their lives and help them in understanding what to do with their time and how to spend it purposefully. Thus, the curriculum content needs to be an extension of what happened in Phase two with three discreet elements developing students' understanding of their life-style. These three discreet elements should provide the opportunity for students to:

- choose an absorbing interest from either a disciplined form of physical activity (eg sport, dance or adventure) or from the alternative activity curriculum from Phase two;

- continue their initiation into a practical knowledge base for their health and well-being;
- take a course which introduces them to a study of life-styles and stimulates discussion about the role of physical activity as one potential choice.

The opportunity to engage in these three elements must be in the context of:

- a negotiated curriculum; and
- student-centred learning;

where the emphasis strengthens a concern for personal development. The roots for such an emphasis started in Phase two when pupils were given the opportunity to learn how to:

- take responsibility for learning; and
- be involved in decision making about their learning and the kind of experiences appropriate to their needs and interests.

This leading in process was part of sport education, the experiential learning of a practical knowledge base for health and well-being, and such activities as the making of a dance and presentation to an audience and the planning of an adventure expedition.

The idea of a negotiated curriculum is a major step forward because if students are to make practical informed choices about their life-style when they leave school they need to learn how to take responsibility for their choices, and teachers need to be aware of students' interests and what 'real' choices students have access to in the community. The process of negotiation will involve taking into account what a student has done in Phase two, what their current interests are and how much involvement they have in such interests, and discussing with the student how a physical education curriculum can be designed with their interests in mind.

A negotiated curriculum will require teachers to make provision for periodic student feedback about their progress, their interests and desires, for careful record keeping of what students have done during their school life, and the opportunity for discussion betwen student and tutors. If it is impossible to accommodate particular interests within the school curriculum, teachers will need to know how these interests can be pursued outside school within community provision or a club and help the student to make contact. Planning a negotiated curriculum will need to start early, because taking student interests and the range of possible combinations into account will require organisational skills to group students with appropriate tutors. This may involve collaboration with staff in other subject areas – for example art, design and music – to consider the provision of student interests, and consultation with timetabling staff to examine the possibilities. For some teachers it may be necessary to acquire timetabling skills in order to devise creative ways of incorporating new organisational patterns that take into account the specific needs of physical education. A modular style curriculum may be able to solve some of these problems, creating new patterns of curriculum organisation.

I do not believe that recreation type courses in the fourth and fifth years of secondary education serve useful purposes and the term option courses associated with them needs to be carefully evaluated. There is some evidence (McNeil, 1987) to show that in the later secondary years there is little relationship between curriculum activities and what young people take part in, or what is available, within the community. Also, the interest in physical activities has begun to decline. Students' interest in health issues increase during this period and there is still much to be learnt about the role of physical activities in promoting personal health. As changes occur in the final two years of compulsory education and the accreditation of courses for GCSE (modular studies), TVEI, B Tech (foundation studies) and records of achievement become a major requirement, I believe it is necessary for physical education to plan courses so that they can be evaluated by out of school agencies and accreditation provided.

Physical education can benefit from this move because accreditation is more than simply an examination course, it is an opportunity to design courses which are part of general education but highlight the specific contribution that our subject can make to life skills, leisure preparation, life-style education, health studies, social skills, social and vocational education, and personal development.

In addition to the negotiated curriculum it is important for teachers to recognise the significance of student-centred learning to assist the transition from school to involvement in physical activity in the community, to cater for the changing needs of students, and contribute to personal development. The roots for such learning began much earlier in Phase two during the middle years of schooling, but now they reach into the very heart of learning in Phase three. With the advent of a restructuring of the 14–18 curriculum, approaches like active tutorial work, supported self-study, experiential learning, active learning, and personal education have involved many teachers in a process of rethinking the way that students are involved in their own learning. In the same way, student-centred learning in physical education has become a focus for many teachers (Matharu, 1987). What is involved in such a focus? I should like to propose the following key components:

- learning from doing;
- sharing in learning;
- ownership of learning; and
- independence.

LEARNING FROM DOING
This involves the use of direct personal experience – an active rather than passive learning process – as the basis for internalising what is to be learnt and thereby acquiring understanding and competence. There is an emphasis on the planning process, prior to 'the doing', and a particular emphasis on the reflection of one's actions to reinforce the internalising process.

SHARING IN LEARNING
This requires the active involvement of students in both what is to be learnt but also the curriculum content to be experienced, and therefore there is a close association with the negotiated curriculum. However, sharing in learning involves also learning with and from others (not just the teacher), so that students are able to respect, be sensitive and tolerant towards different perspectives and the views of others.

OWNERSHIP OF LEARNING
This is a critical aspect which involves a number of key ideas central to student-centred learning. Students need to learn how to set themselves personal goals and strive to achieve them, and in the process make commitments. It means that teachers need to provide the opportunity for students to make personal responses to tasks and challenges, as well as use their imagination

to create something of their own. In these processes the student is learning to assume responsibilities and to be responsible.

INDEPENDENCE
This aspect is about moving from a state of dependence on others (including the teacher) towards independence in the learning process. It involves a recognition that improvement can come as one learns to take control over one's attempts to achieve, and in the process confidence grows providing a new perspective to the learning process.

Conclusions

In this chapter I have attempted to sketch out reasons why physical education should have a place in the education of young people in schools and this has been translated into a framework for the physical education curriculum. This framework provides the basis for teachers to think about the process of constructing a curriculum and to discipline their selection of practical possibilities. However, there are some further considerations to take on board before this process can begin. In the construction of a curriculum teachers do not always receive sufficient time to include all that they would like, therefore, I would like to conclude this article by outlining some further considerations.

Teachers of physical education need to consider how their subject can exist within the whole curriculum. First, physical education has a contribution to make as a unique single subject with its own time allocation. However, this is hardly sufficient, therefore they need to be aware of other ways in which their aspirations can be fulfilled. Second, teachers need to integrate and collaborate with other subject areas. In one sense all subjects are contributing to a general education, like moral and social education, therefore physical education teachers need to be aware of what other subject areas are striving to do and how they contribute to general education. It may be physical education can play such a role, but if time is short this may have to be left alone because it is being adequately covered already. In another way, collaboration with other subject areas may be necessary in health education, performing arts, leisure studies, life style education or life skills. It may also be the case that additional time can be gained by considering GCSE modular studies, TVEI, CPVE, and B Tech (foundation studies) courses as potential avenues for pursuing physical education aspirations. Also, collaboration in terms of organisational needs may create opportunities for a wider choice of potential modules and such liaisons should be pursued with some vigour. Last, the role of physical education as a means of promoting the school should not be overlooked. Events like Healthy Eating Day, the Stress Factor, Health Education Week, and a Heart Day involve a whole school commitment that reinforces physical education's role. Festivals of dance or sport provide the opportunity for the school to become involved with the community. Sporting fixtures and days of dance involve other schools in promoting important educational values, so do school trips and special events. All of these enterprises involve physical education and the fulfilment of important aspirations, but they should not all come out of physical education time. It is important for teachers to plan and reflect how best physical education can translate complex aspirations into a reality within schools.

Notes

1. In the writing of this section I have been influenced strongly by the following writers (Aspin, 1986; Bailey, 1984; Degenhardt, 1982; Warnock, 1978; White, 1982) who have informed my own thoughts and provided me with scope for reflecting on the values of physical education.

References

Alderson, G J K (1982) *Thinking About the PE Curriculum* (pp 2–31) Report of the 2nd Annual Conference of Heads of Departments in Post-Primary Schools. North Eastern Educational and Library Board, Ballymena, Co Antrim.

Arnold, P (1979) *Meaning in Movement, Sport and Physical Education* Heinemann, London.

Aspin, D N (1986) On the nature and purposes of a sporting activity: the connection between sport, life and politics, *Physical Education Review* 9 (1) 5–13.

Bailey, C (1984) *Beyond the Present and the Particular: A Theory of Liberal Education* Routledge & Kegan Paul, London.

Degenhardt, M A B (1982) *Education and the Value of Knowledge* George Allen & Unwin, London.

Dickenson, B (1987) A Survey of the Activity Patterns of Young People and their Attitudes and Perceptions of Physical Activity and Physical

Education in a Local Education Authority unpublished MPhil thesis, Loughborough University of Technology.

Lawton, D (1975) *Class, Culture and the Curriculum* Routledge & Kegan Paul, London.

McNeil, M C (1987) Physical Activity Patterns and Physical Education in Melton Mowbray Schools unpublished project for MSc course, Loughborough University of Technology.

Matharu, J (1987) Student-centred learning. Unpublished document for Health and Physical Education Project, Loughborough University of Technology.

Meakin, D (1986) The moral status of competition: an issue of concern for physical education *Journal of Philosophy of Education* 20 (1), 59–67.

Miller, D M (1988) Scoring ethically in sport *Strategies* 1 (3) 5–7.

Powell, K E and Paffenbarger, R S (1985) Workshop on epidemiologic and public health aspects of physical activity and exercise *Public Health Reports* 100, 118–26.

Skilbeck, M (1984) *School-based Curriculum Development* Harper & Row, London.

Von Wright, G H (1963) *The Varieties of Goodness* Routledge & Kegan Paul, London.

Warnock, M (1978) *Schools of Thought* Faber, London.

Warnock, M (1988) *A Common Policy for Education* Oxford University Press, Oxford.

White, J (1982) *The Aims of Education Restated* Routledge & Kegan Paul, London.

Part 2

Introduction

The chapters in this part home in on traditional activities within physical education and emphasise innovations which have challenged the dominant focus of teachers' work in schools. As innovations they are problematic because of the challenge they represent to traditional thinking, but also, they illustrate how a change of content has implications for relationships with pupils which may indicate a bigger shift of focus in the values of physical education.

The first example of innovation comes from games teaching which takes the lion's share of time in physical education for both boys and girls. This innovation which was called 'teaching for understanding' began slowly in the mid 1970s when it was taught to student-teachers but it only emerged as a significant change of focus for games teaching in the 1980s with the publication of a Bulletin of Physical Education devoted completely to rethinking games. The instigators of this innovation, Thorpe and Bunker, strongly acknowledge the roots of their change of focus which came from the pioneering work of Allen Wade and Eric Worthington in soccer and inspired their own rethinking process. As a result of in-service courses in local education authorities, teaching for understanding emerged as an exciting possibility for changing the focus of all games. However, after a healthy start with articles and courses this innovation began to lose impetus as little material emerged from Loughborough after 1984. The reason for this 'slowing down' represents a major feature of much of our work in physical education and curriculum development. The instigators of teaching for understanding were involved in other innovations, notably sports leadership, and as a consequence their priorities shifted. This is understandable when we rely on developments within an activity emerging only because individuals are prepared to devote time to publicising their work on a national basis.

During the time of the Schools Council when most subject areas received funding to develop new initiatives, physical education was noticeable by its absence. The funding of new initiatives led to the emergence of professional structures which have assisted in the continued development of initiatives at local level. Physical education's absence from the massive curriculum development projects of the late 1960s and 1970s has meant that distinguished practitioners have had to disseminate their work as a sideline and in piecemeal fashion with the slow evaluation of ideas, hardly conducive to the establishment of a firm basis for curriculum development.

However, teaching for understanding was publicised widely and many teachers have attended in-service courses resulting in the growth of articles in professional journals from colleagues in different establishments and schools throughout the country, which demonstrates the impact that this innovation has made. But, when one reads some of these articles and notes the comments published in the ILEA report 'My favourite subject' which came from a working party on school sport chaired by Peter McIntosh, one wonders how messages of innovation are interpreted and assimilated into people's thinking. Teaching for understanding is seen by many of these writers as a way of discussing the tactics of the game, it is interpreted as merely small-sided games or children creating their own games, or something that good teachers have always done.

On reflection, teaching for understanding was probably the wrong term. 'Game-centred games' is more appropriate, but as Thorpe and Bunker clearly show in their chapter the change of focus in games teaching is radically different from the traditional model for presenting games to young people. The way in which they illustrate the essence of games teaching requires close attention and deserves to be properly tested by teachers in practice and not discarded because of an inadequate understanding of what games entail and what they have to offer. Games offer a rich potential for joy and satisfaction through activity, how they are represented to young people is the key to further participation.

Bob Smith's analysis of the changing emphasis within gymnastics and his summary of the conflicts that split the physical education profession provides a timely reminder of the problems of innovation and the reality of translating a complex idea into practical teaching proposals that teachers can absorb. His analysis of the current changing focus or restatement of direction illustrates how important it is to establish a clear framework to guide practice and discipline teachers' actions in schools. However, such a framework is only beginning to emerge and the gymnastics world needs to learn from the work on games teaching that many practical exemplars are essential if teachers are to assimilate and accommodate ideas and put them into practice. Knowing the rhetoric of innovation will not guarantee success. However, Bob Smith's chapter offers hope because there is the will to work together and the inspiration of John Wright to make the translation of ideas a practical possibility. The gymnastics chapter introduces the notion of teaching styles which has influenced a number of people in institutes of higher education during the past five years. It provides a useful heuristic for developing ideas, but it needs to be treated as an insight into a range of possibilities rather than received wisdom and a path that has to be followed. Hence the need for teachers to be critical consumers of innovation. These ideas can discipline our thinking and inform our perspectives but they must remain a heuristic as ideas begin to develop and grow.

Colin Hardy's presentation of an integrated approach to swimming provides us with a comprehensive analysis of how teachers can logically plan the development of swimming in schools. His model takes the teacher step-by-step through a gradual progression of potential swimming experiences. This kind of planning provides the teacher with one way of mapping how an activity can be planned and implemented, and therefore it has implications for other aspects of physical education. When teachers are increasingly required to submit their planning to scrutiny and accreditation, Hardy's model can provide teachers with clear guidelines for action.

The chapter on athletics demonstrates how a change of focus – in the way that we recognise success – has important implications for all young people in schools. The use of a classification scheme to guide the selection of activities that pupils will experience provides a more comprehensive range of athletic challenges than those currently in vogue. It is interesting to note that the use of the term 'material of athletics' and the idea of 'action possibilities' are similar to those used in gymnastics. John Wright's work in gymnastics was a powerful inspiration for the origin of the athletics classification scheme and illustrates how much we can learn from each other in translating the essence of an activity – like athletics – into a framework for action which disciplines what is taught.

Finally, Bryan Smith raises a host of issues in his analysis of developments in outdoor education and residential experiences. During the past few years changes have been taking place in such a way that outdoor education has associated itself with different partners within a school. Also, the elitism of some approaches to outdoor pursuits has led many people to look at alternative ways of presenting adventure challenges to young people in the local environment and around the school. These developments provide tremendous scope. Teachers of physical education have yet to recognise this and grasp the significance of these changes for a re-focus within the current physical education curriculum. Bryan Smith introduces us to an aspect of personal and social development which forms a major part of recent initiatives within outdoor education. In many respects this aspect has received more attention in outdoor education than in any other area of physical education. Teachers can learn much from their approach in the preparation of guidelines to highlight this crucial area of a child's development.

At this point the reader will have noticed the absence of dance from this section on innovations within physical education. This is quite deliberate because much of the dance world has been moving over into performing arts, a movement that I find myself in agreement with. The reduction of time for physical education in the curriculum will mean that dance work will suffer. Also, the profession has failed to persuade its male members to recognise the significance of a dance experience for all boys and as a consequence many boys do not have the opportunity to engage in any sort of meaningful encounter with dance. The movement towards a health focus within physical education will mean that some teachers will use dance time to introduce exercise to music and neglect important aspects of dance work. However, the rationalisaton of time in the curriculum will inevitably mean that physical education will suffer and as a consequence there will be much debate about what constitutes physical education. Already some teachers in anticipation of such a reduction have found exciting ways of developing particular aspects of physical education in areas like the CPVE framework and TVEI. The GCSE dance course has proved to be very successful, therefore I believe that dance can learn to exist in its own right for all pupils and stand alongside traditional academic courses.

The developments within physical education at the present moment need some form of urgent rationalisation, because without this, piecemeal initiatives will be added on to existing structures to form an unwieldy amalgam. It is in this context that dance has a better chance of survival and room for future growth. However hard this decision may sound realistic assessments have to be made.

Chapter 2
A Changing Focus in Games Teaching

Rod Thorpe and David Bunker

Introduction

Throughout the 1970s an approach to teaching games was formulated which placed the emphasis on ensuring that children understood the games they played while capitalising on the intrinsic motivation most youngsters bring towards playing the game. It is interesting to note that we use the phrase 'playing the game' but we do not use the phrases 'playing athletics' or 'playing swimming'. The problem seems to have been that a number of teachers found it difficult to resolve the relationship between the game and game skills.

Clearly to play a game well the skills have to be well-practised and it is logical to give children as much skill practice as possible. The major problem with this approach is that we (and many teachers we discovered later) realised that for many children the time available in the curriculum was insufficient to perfect or even reach adequate levels with many of the games skills, particularly, if the teacher was always teaching the average child. The less able were forced to recognise their inadequacies and the very able went unchallenged. The whole class waited for the game, particularly in those lessons based on the quite common format of an introduction and a technique/skill, followed a game. Of course, teachers taught through the game and conditioned practices but by their own admission did not really have a clear philosophy or framework within which to work. This problem seems to be international if the comment made in the introduction to our article, presented in the *South Australian PE Bulletin* in 1984, is typical:

> ... the idea of progressing from tactics to skills, or from Why? to How? rather than vice versa, is not new, but its organisation and application has not previously been made coherent.

The interchange with students, teachers, advisers and our colleagues led us to propose a model which was first published in the *Bulletin of Physical Education* (1982). The model, shown in Figure 2.1, is central to the way we plan lessons and/or units of work and indeed helps us to formulate an overall programme. It is included here by way of introduction.

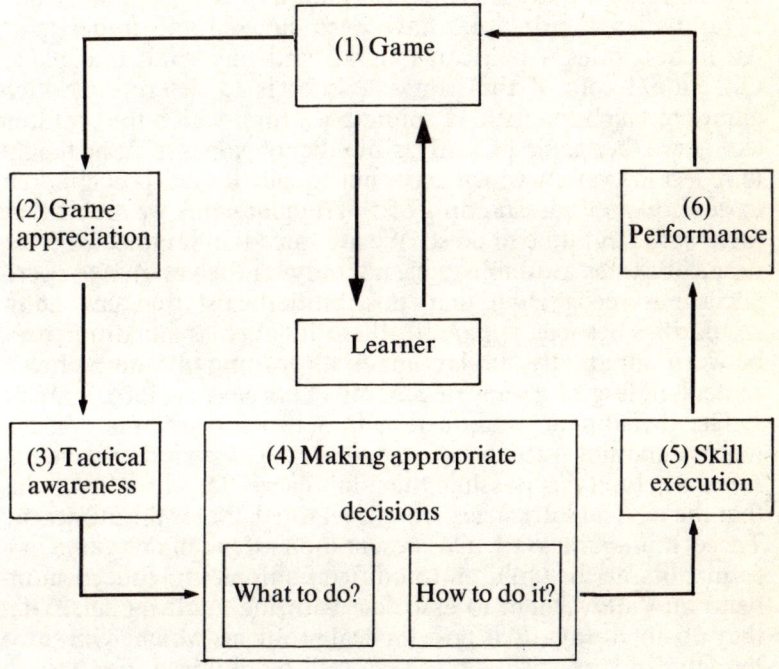

Figure 2.1   *Model for games teaching*

It is important to recognise that while the approach stresses understanding, that understanding is incomplete if it is not done in the practical situation. The overt sign that understanding has been fully gained is some form of appropriate response.

It may be idealistic (and why not?) to hope that we can educate future generations who can watch games on the television and understand the basic tactics involved.

Thorpe *et al* (1986) have discussed the idea that we can develop a games curriculum based on this model coupled with four fundamentals:

- sampling;
- modification – representation;
- modification – exaggeration;
- tactical complexity.

In our experience the person who really understands the game of soccer can appreciate what players are trying to do in a hockey game and is certainly not completely unaware of basketball tactics. If fundamental principles have been stressed and understood, Australian rules, American football and rugby fall into place. One initial role of the games teacher is to determine which games to teach to ensure a sound base from which the children can view other games. Clearly, a number of games must be taught to reflect the variety which exists but equally if we expect children to develop an understanding of a particular game we must allow them sufficient time to do so. We are forced to 'sample' from the range of games available to us, not only for the variety of experiences but recognising that 'possibilities exist that can show similarities between apparently dissimilar games and differences between apparently similar games, all leading to a much better understanding of games in general' (Thorpe *et al*, 1986, p. 164).

The division of modification into two fundamentals is not mere semantics – teachers can modify a game so that it 'represents' as closely as possible the adult game. This usually means that the tactical intricacies are still retained, that is the attraction. These 'mini-games' are a 'representation' of the major game in a form suitable for children (modified equipment, reduced numbers) and allow them to associate with the adult model. What they do not always do is pose tactical problems which, with some thought and practice, can be 'solved' by children. For this to happen elements of the games have to be exaggerated. A 'thin' badminton court which makes it obvious that the space to attack is at the front and back of the court is an example of exaggeration.

If the aim is to ensure that children understand the games they play it would seem logical to start with the simpler games. In fact, we find 11-a-side soccer being taught to nine-year-olds while the tactically less complex game of 1 *v* 1 badminton or tennis is left until 14 years of age. With the development of modified games and the availability of sufficient equipment it becomes far more realistic to present the tactically simple games first, which would seem to be a sensible procedure.

These four fundamentals will be used to develop a 5–16 curriculum, because they provide a framework of principles to guide our practice.

Games in the primary school

It is of course ironic that while most physical education specialists recognise that the 5–11 year period is vital for physical development few specialists work in this area. This has often resulted in a very limited games experience in the primary school. It might be useful to consider four approaches to games which are or could be seen in the primary school.

First, the physical education lesson consists of movement/ gymnastics/dance/or relays, and the children have a separate games lesson in which the children play seven-a-side netball, 11-a-side soccer and, when it is warm, 9-a-side rounders with the teacher as the feeder. Of course we feel that this is quite inappropriate, the children get few chances to use skills learnt and there is little chance of children understanding the games they play.

Second, the physical education lesson is as above but when it comes to the games, teachers use 'mini' forms of the adult game eg 4 v 4 netball with players allowed to go anywhere on their court except that only the two attackers can go in the other team's semi-circle and only the two defenders can go in their own semi-circle. A general agreement that all primary schools will play mini-games in lessons and in school matches would improve the games experience dramatically. Selecting one or two 'mini' invasion games such as 4 v 4 netball or 5 v 5 soccer/rugby/ hockey, a court game or two (eg 3 v 3 volleyball or short tennis) or a small sided fielding game like 5 v 5 rounders or cricket, would ensure a more varied and more valuable game experience (we think). Even so we are not convinced that the problems set by these games are clear enough for the children to find solutions to them.

Third, it can be argued that traditional games have been developed for adults by adults and that merely reducing them to 'mini games' is still not moving far enough if children are to really understand. It may be far better to choose and/or design games specifically to suit children at this stage of their learning and development.

Fourth, the recognition that games should be designed for children leads quite naturally to the idea that children can be allowed to design and develop their own games within confines set by the teacher. The area of games making, particularly when used with a well-structured programme, and not as an excuse for the teacher's failure to think about games, can help children to understand the need for rules and simple tactics.

Finally, if one believes that the underlying central theme of a games education is to build up an understanding of how to play games, it goes without saying that whatever games are selected they should be arranged in an order which allows the development of this understanding. It may be necessary to move from one set of games to another if this is to be achieved.

FOR PRIMARY SCHOOL INFANTS (5–7)

A pupil throws the ball somewhere specific – a simple target game occurs – 'can I hit that "object"?'

A friend joins in and we start to count – 'I'll have five goes, then you have five goes.' 'How many did we get together?' 'I beat you.' At this stage we may start to help children to 'compete' with care.

The teacher encourages the children to aim for different sorts of target, a hoop on the floor, a circle on the wall, a bucket etc.

The partner becomes a target who has to catch the ball without moving. Here, we are still playing target games.

FOR JUNIORS (7–11)

One throws the ball at a big target – the other tries to stop it hitting the target. The target on the wall might now look like a goal. The target on the floor might now be a court. The children learn to throw away from the goalkeeper or fielder, who finds out how to defend the area (Figure 2.2).

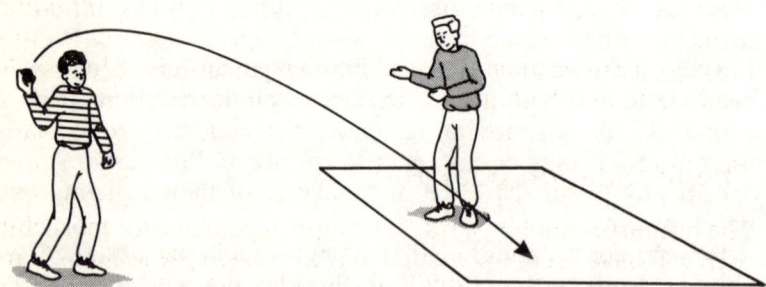

Figure 2.2 *Children bowling towards and defending a target*

From this point we could let two children work together to defend the area against the thrower; now they are involved in a fielding game.

Having ensured that the children are now clear on how to attack a space and how to defend it, they can be moved to alternate rapidly between attack and defence by playing a divided court game (Figure 2.3).

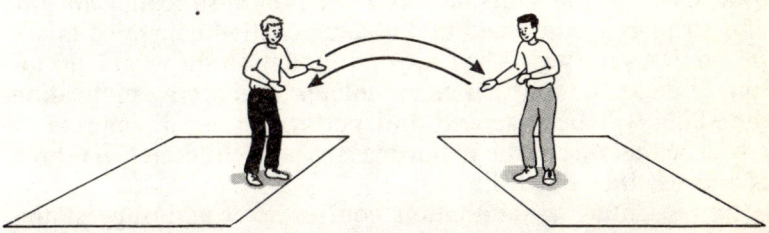

Figure 2.3 *Alternate attacking and defending*

With two squares an appropriate distance apart and perhaps a large sponge ball, we can play throw catch tennis or badminton.

Putting a high net between the two courts and introducing another two players we can move from 1 *v* 1 towards a 2 *v* 2 throw volleyball-type game.

Put the net away, put the children into threes, each three in their own square, and play 'piggy in the middle'; the piggy is like the net but of course she/he can move – we have taken the first step towards 4 *v* 4 invasion games mentioned previously.

At any stage the teacher can move off into a more recognisable game, eg 1 *v* 1 throw tennis becomes 1 *v* 1 short tennis if a bat is used, but perhaps only after the 2 *v* 2 fielding game so that the youngsters get used to using the bat with a friend feeding them.

For us the ideal primary games programme would lead children through games which become increasingly complex, leaning heavily on throw-catch games at first which allow the children to catch, hold and look: they often need that time to think.

The foundation course

The primary school physical education experience for most children will have been limited to playing invasion games, which are without doubt the most difficult games to play. Whether it be on a scaled-down football pitch or on a small size netball court, the skills involved in receiving the ball, controlling it and directing the pass, with an opponent, sometimes more than one, breathing down the neck, are much too demanding for all but a very few. In the light of their 'poor skills' some children find themselves practising 'ball skills' in the first year of their secondary school games course. While such courses may be of some help, it is inevitable that much of the work is based on techniques with next to no time spent on playing games. We see little justification for this and strongly recommend that a game-centred course be taught in the first year which lays a firm foundation for what is to follow. If the games chosen create interest and strong motivation, the skills will be practised and performance will improve. It could be that one of the major reasons why children can't throw is because they don't throw.

In presenting a foundation course we would suggest that teachers start a 2 *v* 2 striking–fielding game. The more controlled tempo within such games can be a real advantage: the striker is free to choose when and where to hit the ball and need not be too concerned with what happens next. The ball will not come straight back from the other side and nobody is going to get close enough to interfere with the strike. To get the striking-fielding game going we need to change the bat and ball and make sure that the striker and pitcher – becoming a co-operative feeder – are on the same side. In so doing skill thresholds are reduced and we stand a much better chance of keeping players, particularly the fielders, more involved. It should be said that there is no place in such a foundation course for the 'traditional' games of 'rounders' or 'cricket' . . . elsewhere maybe.

A 2 *v* 2 game can be played quite conveniently on an area the size of a badminton court. The fielders defend half the court while the strike is made from anywhere behind the baseline. This is shown in Figure 2.4.

The striker can choose whether to self-feed or to receive a 'friendly' throw from the pitcher. Any striking implement can be used and any kind of soft ball, a padder bat and a sponge tennis ball make an interesting combination. In the early stages some youngsters should be allowed to throw the ball into the fielding area if they so wish. To complete an innings both players have six hits each – one point is given if the ball crosses the line at halfway, two for the sidelines and four for the backline but the ball *must bounce* in the fielding area.

A good deal of teaching material stems from this simple game

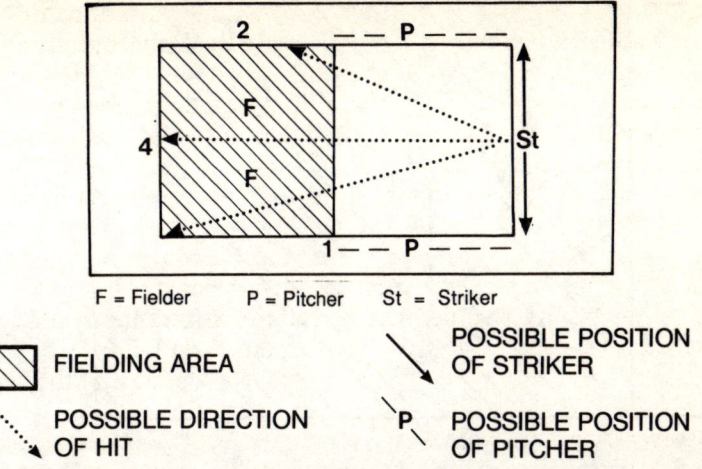

F = Fielder   P = Pitcher   St = Striker

▨ FIELDING AREA

⬊ POSSIBLE POSITION OF STRIKER

⋰⬏ POSSIBLE DIRECTION OF HIT

ˋP̖ POSSIBLE POSITION OF PITCHER

Figure 2.4   *2 v 2 game showing striking and defending areas*

situation. Particular lessons might take account of the following points:

- How is the striker coming to terms with the problem of making the ball bounce in the fielding area? Is (s)he hitting from high to low? or bending down to hit a 'skimmer' . . . or sending the ball along the floor? Is the ball being hit hard or being placed into an open space? Is there any use of spin, angles and disguise?
- Where do the fielders take up position at the start of the game? Are they standing side by side, at front or back, or are they fielding one behind the other? Why do they field in these positions? Which fielder takes responsibility for the space down the middle? What is the most effective way of stopping the ball?

Over the last few years we have built a basic 3 *v* 3 game into our work on a foundation course. The format of the game is quite different from the 2 *v* 2 set up, the striker is confronted with an unusual task and much more is asked of the fielders (Figure 2.5).

The striker hits three balls, one after the other (or simultaneously) into the fielding area and then runs round the bases (of course there is no reason why the balls should not be thrown or kicked into the fielding area). Meanwhile the fielders retrieve the balls and return them as quickly as possible to any two of the

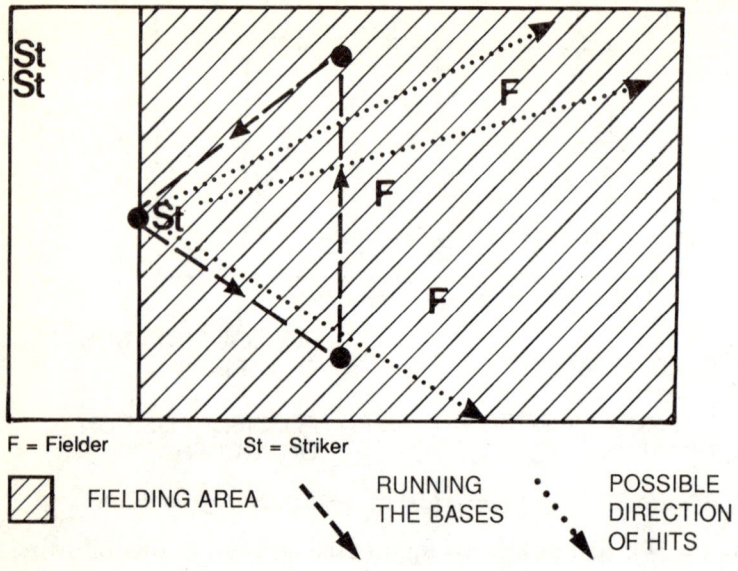

F = Fielder   St = Striker

FIELDING AREA   RUNNING THE BASES   POSSIBLE DIRECTION OF HITS

Figure 2.5 *3 v 3 game using more than one ball*

bases before the striker completes the 'home run'. Points can be awarded for reaching first and second bases.

The striker must decide when, where and how to hit the balls. Is it best to launch them in rapid fire, or to delay the third hit momentarily? Should the hits be directed at any one fielder? Might it be a good idea to play all three balls into the close field or should they be hit high and deep into the back field?

With so many options available to the striker, the fielders will have plenty to think about. First and foremost they will have to work as a team. Where should the field be set? Is it better for two fielders to cover the deep field? Who is going to receive the ball on the bases? Should one of the fielders run one ball to a base instead of throwing it? Planning for every eventuality is going to take some time!

Too often we see striking–fielding games being played in which there is too little activity. After waiting some time for a hit, few youngsters make a good contact (or any contact) with the ball which, in turn, means that the fielders are made redundant. This should not be allowed to happen in the foundation course, or, we would add, in later years.

The following is but one example of a game which keeps every-

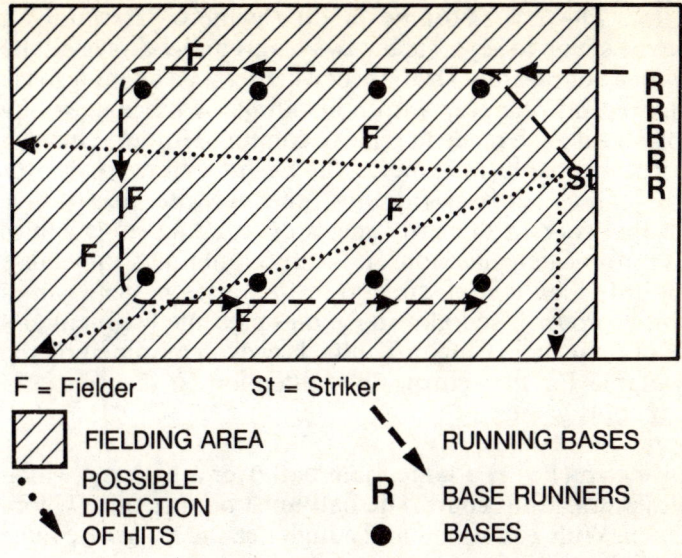

F = Fielder   St = Striker

FIELDING AREA   RUNNING BASES

POSSIBLE
DIRECTION   R   BASE RUNNERS
OF HITS

●   BASES

Figure 2.6 *Active striking–fielding game*

one on their toes and which requires those taking part, especially
the fielders, to think about the tactics used (Figure 2.6).

The game starts with a self-feed and a strike into the fielding
area. One of the fielders recovers the ball and sends it to base 1
from where it is transferred round the bases to finish at base 8.
As soon as the hit is made, the striker sets off closely followed by
others in the team, to complete a run round the bases. The fact
that everyone on the striking side runs the bases after every hit
makes this a demanding game for them as well as the fielders.
The game gives plenty of scope for introducing different scoring
systems. The tactics developed in response to changes in the
scoring will give an indication of the understanding of the different games being played. Whatever else may happen, the striker
will have to decide where best to hit the ball – 'as far away from
the first base as possible' – a good tactic if the rule states that the
ball must be relayed from first base . . . and the fielders will have
to come together to decide on their individual responsibilities for
retrieving the ball and covering the bases as well as the best
means of transforming the ball from base to base . . . it could
depend on the type of ball being used.

It does not take much to step out of a fielding game into a

court game. The 2 v 2 striking–fielding game only requires a barrier to be set up to separate the two teams and we have all the makings of a court game. The barrier whether it be a line, a space or a net, prevents one player from invading the other's territory and allows a hit to be made in relative comfort. However, in such games, it is probable that there will be little time to recover before the ball comes back from the other side. Because of this, much of the work in the early stages of teaching court games explores throw–catch situations. It is important that a rally takes place for only then is it possible to further a youngster's games education on court. The following games presented sequentially in terms of their increasing difficulty, largely determined by the time available for the return, draw attention to the dos (and don'ts) of court games.

1. Throw-catch (1 v 1) a large foam ball over a high net which divides a long, thin court. The ball must bounce once before the catch. With a slow ball and a high net, the rallies are long, there is plenty of time to execute the throw.

   Points to note. The importance of throwing to the baseline to keep the opponent as far away from the net as possible. It is much easier to win the point from close to the net.

2. The same 1 v 1 game but with a rule change: the ball must not bounce.

   Points to note. Continue to throw long, wait for an opportunity to win the point, ie your opponent is out of position at the back of the court. Drop the ball over the net into the space at the front of the court.

3. Add another rule to the same 1 v 1 game: the ball must be thrown from the catch position.

   Points to note. Make every effort to catch the ball at its highest point; throwing from below the height of the net will give both the time and the opportunity for your opponent to make a winning return. Remember that to throw (or hit) from low to high is to defend.

   After each throw recover quickly to the point on the court which helps you defend the court.

4. A 2 v 2 passing game introduces the element of team play

and could bring the hit into the game: one of the players, after making a catch, throws the ball for the other to hit over the net. It is a good idea to let the second player decide on whether to catch and throw or whether to hit over the net. To keep the rally going, the advantage to be gained from the hits on one side of the net is offset by allowing the ball to bounce once on the other side.

Points to note. The first catcher takes aim to make sure that the ball is 'set' high in the front court, near to the net. The other player prepares to hit or throw down into the opponents' court.

From here a 3 *v* 3 game requiring a catch–throw, a throw, and a hit from both teams is not far removed from the 'dig', 'set' and 'spike' sequence of the game of volleyball.

With some idea as to how to play a good tactical game and with some experience of hitting the ball, albeit with the hand, we might now introduce a padder bat and a small, slow ball to facilitate the 'hit–hit' sequence of the more traditional court games. In retaining the one bounce rule and a high net, it is hoped that rallies will develop and that many, if not all, of the points made in the throw–catch games will be transferred to this modified game of padder tennis. As things improve, ie the rallies become more prolonged, other changes, notably lowering the net, bringing the volley into play, introducing a short tennis racket, can be made. At the end of the foundation course on court games, it would be most reassuring to watch rallies in which deep approach shots were opening up the court for winning vollies. It would be even more reassuring to see a good approach shot met with an equally good defensive lob, a recovery to make another approach shot to force a more shallow lob and a winning smash. It is clear that each shot is being played to good purpose and shows a well-developed tactical understanding of the changing circumstances of the rally.

We would start our work in the invasion games by playing 'pig in the middle', a game well known to 11-year-olds. The 2 *v* 1 situation is fundamental in the teaching of invasion games. An instruction to 'keep the ball for 30 seconds' (keepball) might result in the youngster with the ball doing very little except hold on to it! Great! . . . but the defender might not allow this to happen if a decision is made to attack the ball. But now the defender has been drawn towards the ball, space has been created and the pass can be made more safely. In getting the receiver to take up good positions, some time (and not a little effort) will be necessary to establish the need to move off the ball, to move away from the ball more often, perhaps, than towards it, to change direction and to provide the best possible passing angle. Another instruction 'to make as many passes as possible in 30 seconds' (speedball) puts a much greater burden on the receiver. A thinking defender will mark one player only who when passing and receiving will find it difficult to create space, but does it matter if the pass is not made as long as the ball can be recovered quickly for another attempt? However, if a penalty of three points is incurred for an incomplete pass it should make the player in possession think twice before releasing the ball. The risk might be too great, if so the ball will be held to wait for a better passing opportunity. The calculation of risk and safety in attacking (and defending) a variety of targets, some stationary, others moving, some wide, some narrow, is fundamental to an appreciation and understanding of invasion games. The juxtaposition of the two games 'keepball' (30 s.) and 'speedball' (many passes) shows quite clearly how a simple rule change alters the game quite dramatically and causes the thinking player to respond differently to the task.

In developing the work further, we have tended to introduce a game along the lines of skittleball. At first few rules are prescribed – as youngsters see the need for a rule it can be incorporated into the game – usually a passing game emerges in which there is no contact, a 'no-go' area around the target, no travelling and no running with the ball. Points are scored for hitting the skittle. How are we going to make our attack? We must move the ball quickly to the target, if an interception is made it might be worth the risk to take a long shot to penetrate to the target. The defence might try to guard against the 'fast break' by making sure that one player delays the pass or shot by attacking the ball carrier while the others recover to concentrate (or zone) around the skittle. On the other hand defenders might decide to mark man for man to increase the likelihood of regaining possession quickly and to keep the opposition penned in their own half. Decisions such as this must be explored through principles of play and taken in the context of the rules for the game.

For some time (and long before American football became popular in this country) we have played a game that we call 'lineball' to contrast with 'skittleball'. Instead of playing on a long narrow pitch the game is played across so that the 'end' line being attacked is wide (in marked contrast to the narrow goal of skittleball). A score is made by either running with the ball in possession over the line into a large 'end' zone or by throwing the ball into this end zone to be received by a team-mate. A run comes to a halt if a defender manages to tag the runner – the ball must now be thrown with the possibility that possession may be lost (notice that possession is not surrendered despite the tag). This rule is intended to encourage youngsters to run forward with the ball. Very few of them, given their first taste of rugby football, make a forward move. Once they are forced into passing backwards the ball usually finishes behind their own goal line. In giving all the advantages to the attacking team, the defenders must feed off the scraps. The intended receiver may drop the ball, the defender may knock the ball away or better still make an interception, if so, the pass is incomplete and the defending team wins possession. The defenders will need some time to work out the most effective way to protect their line – some form of one-on-one marking will be necessary to stop the run, hopefully before it starts. It might pay dividends to leave one player at least to mark space in a 5 v 5 game. It might be the right thing to do if one team has more players than another but we do not know for certain. The important thing is to find out what works, when it works and why it works. And, of course, while this is going on, we take every opportunity to draw attention to what was covered in 2 v 1, 3 v 1 situations – drawing an opponent, disguising the pass, making an angle, calculating the risks etc.

You cannot spend too much time in planning the foundation course because it is fundamental to a games education and it contains the building blocks for later work in the recognised games.

As part of the foundation course, 'games making', started in the primary school, should be continued and some of the ideas gleaned from children's games will contain many of the ingredients of the 'real' game and, as such, will require that some time be given to find ways round the problems that the game presents. If we teach games, with understanding as a clear objective, supported by the content suggested, the foundation course might capture the interest of a large majority of the youngsters in their first year of the PE curriculum.

From the foundation course to a specific game

CRICKET

In making the move from the foundation course into a more 'recognised' game, it is helpful to refer to the 2 *v* 2 fielding game described previously. With a padder bat, the striker directs the hit towards a pre-determined target area having been 'fed' by a co-operative server. The fielder's plan their tactics, make decisions on the positions to take up, adjust the positions if necessary, work out the angles and hopefully, stop the ball. It is but a short step into a game which looks a little like cricket. With a cricket bat and tennis ball now to hand, the striker (batter) faces the co-operative feeder (bowler) to receive a throw which allows for a good, strong hit to a target area on the 'leg-side' of the striker (Figure 2.7).

The feeder and striker must work together to find the sort of delivery which can be despatched most easily to the target (fielding) area. It should not be too long before most 12/13-year-olds come up with the answer: a ball, bouncing about half-way, aimed at the body and arriving at waist height . . . the bounce gives time to prepare for the shot which is made at a comfortable height. But what sort of shot? Let them work it out. It would be

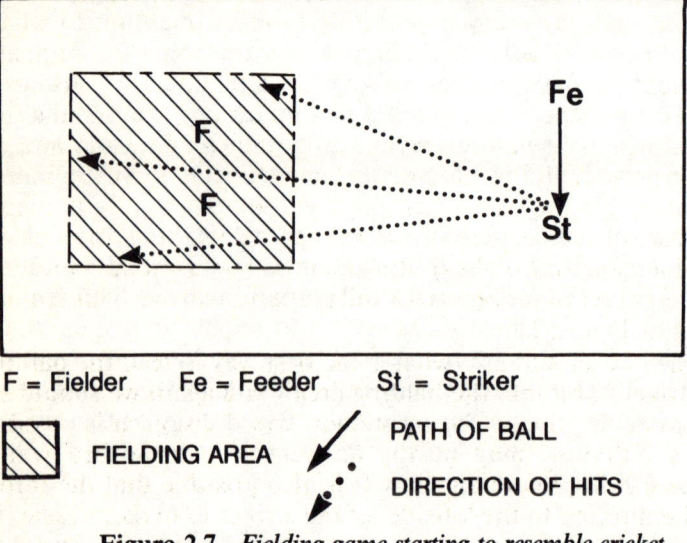

F = Fielder   Fe = Feeder   St = Striker

FIELDING AREA

PATH OF BALL

DIRECTION OF HITS

Figure 2.7 *Fielding game starting to resemble cricket*

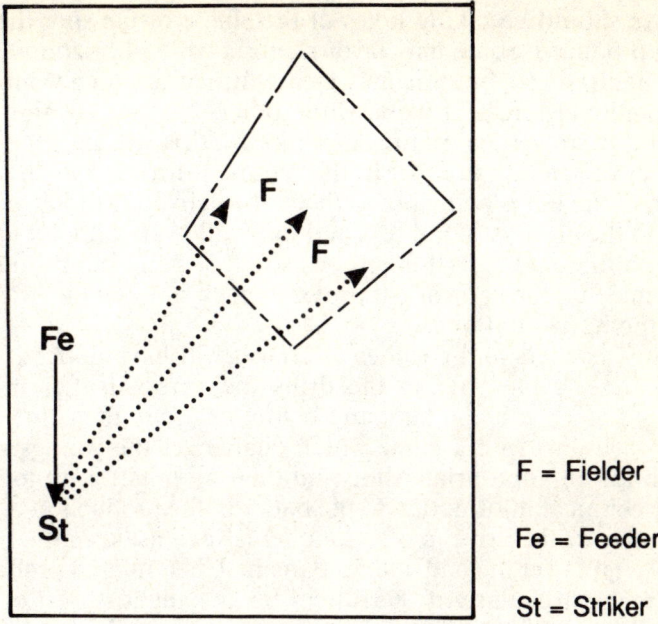

Figure 2.8 *Consequences of altering target area*

surprising if most youngsters were not playing something akin to the 'pull shot' after some trial and error practice. A good contact should be well rewarded as this is a strong hitting action using muscles of the legs and trunk as well as long arms . . . and worth the risk of using a striking surface no more than 4¼ in deep. Including a rule which requires the batter to hit the ball down on to the ground in the fielding area before a run can be scored demands that the pull shot is played from high to low, the more so if it has been decided to reward the fielders for taking a catch. A re-location and slight readjustment to the target area presents a different set of problems for the players involved. This is illustrated in Figure 2.8.

Again we should ask 'what is the best way to feed the ball for the striker to hit into the fielding area?' and again we should set time aside for discussion, negotiation and decision. It is possible that a 'full toss' may be the answer or a throw-feed which bounces twice before arriving. It is also possible that the throw will be directed to the 'offside' of the striker to make it easier to hit into the fielding area. As youngsters find out the best ways to

57

feed we should be taking notes of the shape of the shot that is being produced. Some may favour hitting with a horizontal bat, quite naturally so, but this may create difficulties on account of the rotational forces at work, while others may be keeping the bat in a more vertical plain. As we know, this will increase the chances of sending the ball in the required direction as the full length of the bat is being put to the ball – deliveries which arrive close to the ground, ie full toss and half volley are difficult to hit with a horizontal bat. (It might be as well to point out for future reference that the vertical bat protects much more of the 'wicket' than the horizontal one.)

Many teachers and coaches of cricket will have noticed how close these 'games' are to the drills they present after initial teaching of a particular shot and before its use in the game. But we always start with a game which challenges the youngster to search for an appropriate shot, and then we might want to give some technical information to the batter in the production of the pull to leg or the drive to off. Comments such as 'keep the head still', 'weight over the ball' are fundamental, helpful and probably sufficient, particularly if the rule of being caught is part of the game. It should be remembered that technical advice is given only when it is needed and it is always appropriate to the individual concerned.

So far little has been said about the fielders; of course, every opportunity wil have been taken to reinforce material from the foundation course, but it is a fact that they are dependent upon what is happening between the bowler and the batter . . . with the bowler feeding accurately and the batter striking consistently and with the purpose of penetrating the field, the fielders come more into the picture. The game shown in Figure 2.9 brings them to the centre of the stage.

The rules might be:

- no runs scored unless the ball is hit into the fielding area;
- the ball must be kept below head height for runs to be scored;
- the batter scores 'one', 'two' or 'four' if the ball crosses the appropriate boundary line;
- two bonus runs are scored if batter completes a 'run' between the wickets; and
- the batter is penalised, eg loses a life, loses runs, if 'caught' or 'run out'. (The batter is not out unless a pre-determined number of deliveries have been received or a certain number of runs have been scored.)

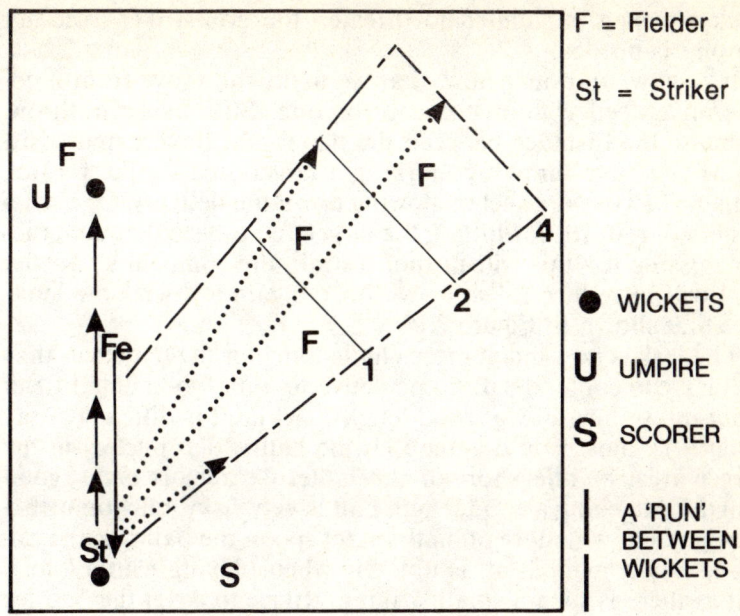

Figure 2.9 *Game providing central role for fielders*

From the outset, a game-centred approach requires that officials will be needed (part of the games education), thus in this game the 'umpire' judges the run-out as laid down in the laws of cricket and the scorer plays a vital part.

It will not have gone unnoticed that decision-making plays a much greater part in this game, more options are available to the striker: 'shall I attack the ball and try for a four?'; 'should I place the ball short and go for a run?', 'should I risk the run?'; 'perhaps I should play safe?' Well, it all depends . . . what is the score? how many are needed to win? how many deliveries are left? where are the fielders placed? . . . The fielders will need to be alert to the different possibilities.

When it is apparent that an intelligent game is being played in the sense that they know what they should be trying to do, and are trying to do it, further progress can be made. The addition of another batter at the umpire's wicket makes the completion of a run much more difficult – running between the wickets is brought into sharp focus. Another fielder, later to function as a wicket-keeper, is situated to threaten the non-striker. Another umpire is needed.

It is now, and only now, that we make the move from a co-operative feeder to a competitive one. Still using a throw, increase the distance between the batter and bowler and insist on an accurate throw by marking a target area for the bowler. This will have the effect of slowing down the delivery. Operate a system of rewards for hitting the target and a system of penalties for missing it – this will further restrain the competitive bowler and will introduce a 'game' within the game which now looks like that shown in Figure 2.10.

The task is now much more challenging for the batters as they will have to contend with some deliveries on a 'good length'. But what do we mean by a 'good length?' While it is difficult to say what it is, most would agree that the ball which pitches in the target area, a little short of the batter's reach, is on a 'good length'. Attacking a good length ball is very risky, playing with a 'straight' bat will more often than not spoon the ball into the air, while any contact at all is unlikely when playing with a 'cross' bat as there is such a small striking surface to cover the bounce of the ball. But the option to play defensively by placing the ball into a space and calling for a run is still available. However, if the bowler is pitching consistently on a good length, the fielders will be able to move in to threaten the run. A very tactical game of 5 v 5 cricket is now under way.

Until now the ball has been delivered by means of a throw, now might be the time to introduce youngsters to the 'bowl'. While they should 'have a go' at developing a basic bowling action few of them will be able to establish sufficient control to bowl with the accuracy needed to challenge the batter and to keep the fielders meaningfully involved. For this reason we should be wary of placing too much importance on being able to bowl. In any case, if the rules of Australian indoor cricket, a game rapidly growing in popularity in this country, allow the bowler to deliver the ball underarm from halfway between the wickets, then why can't we do the same in the PE lesson? Perhaps teachers should take a good look at the various forms of indoor cricket being played (in fact the rules relating to scoring runs in the small side games just described are part and parcel of these games). They do contain some interesting ways in which the game can be shaped in future physical education lessons. It is envisaged in later courses that games will be played in which

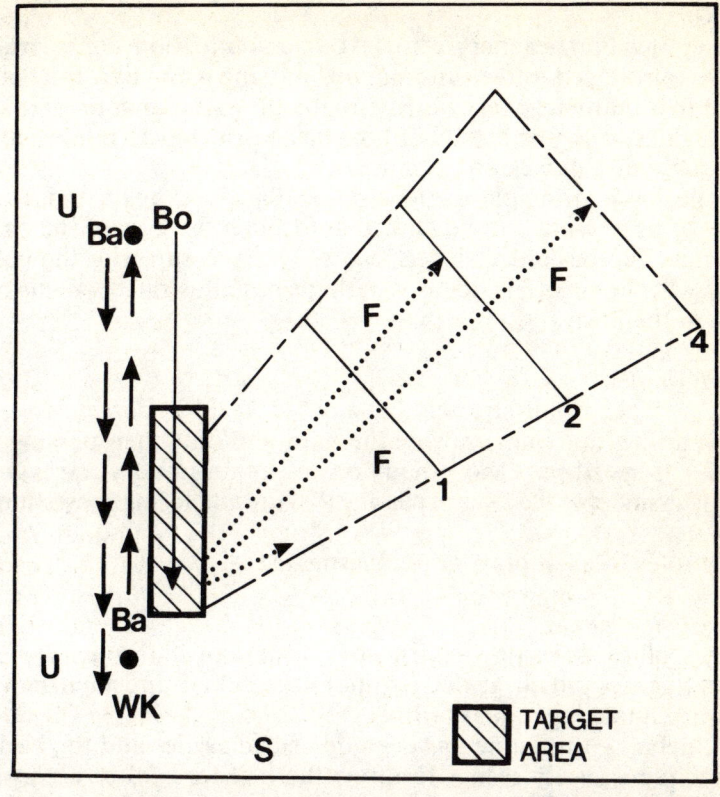

Ba = Batter   Wk = Wicket Keeper   F = Fielder
Bo = Bowler   U = Umpire   S = Scorer

Figure 2.10 *Effect on the game of controlled 'bowling'*

the batter, increasing the range of shots, is allowed to hit the ball all around the wicket; the fielders, in weighing up the costs and benefits of deploying attacking and defending fields, continue to react to the changing circumstances of the game, and the bowler, in trying to dismiss the batter, is introduced to the notion of 'bowling to the field' . . . but not with a hard cricket ball.

61

RUGBY

Accepting that teachers who favour a foundation course will have introduced a free running, free passing game like 'lineball' and that many teachers starting rugby play similar sorts of lead up games, it is worth tracing how basic principles are revisited throughout a games programme.

The basic principle of penetration balanced against risk of loss of possession can be looked at through the eyes of the ball carrier. The basic decision is that of when to run with the ball and when to pass. The focus is perhaps best illustrated by returning to the basics.

Early games
1. 2 *v* 1 keep ball stresses the ways of keeping possession by running, dodging, drawing the man and only then passing.
2. 2 *v* 1 speed pass (how many passes in a minute) stresses the assessment of the risks of passing to score and losing possession.

The roles of each player are investigated.

Developing games
Clearly these roles and the risks can be developed through 2 *v* 2, 4 *v* 4 games which at first are non-directional and then move toward attacking a goal or line.

Lineball – this game has been described earlier and the basic principle is easily seen – to throw the ball forward to a player well down the field penetrates but takes time and because the ball leaves the hands possession might be lost. A run might only make a short penetration but there is no risk of losing possession (Figure 2.11).

Is this so different from the fly half's 'kick or pass' decision in rugby or the quarter back's close pass to a running back or long pass to a wide receiver?

Of course there is so much more to be learnt in lineball but let us merely take the ball carrier's decision into rugby.

Rugby football is an excellent game for highlighting the relative risks and benefits in running with the ball and keeping possession or kicking with resultant ground gained but possession risked. It is these decisions that make rugby exciting and interesting but of course the game must be simplified if this is to be investigated. After many years of teaching and coaching and perhaps, more importantly, trying to help others teach rugby, one of us (Rod

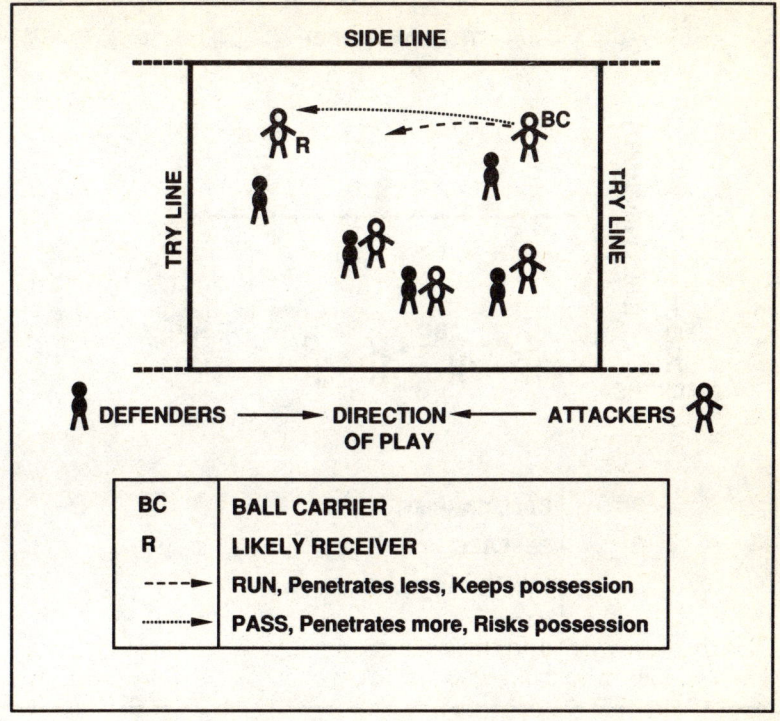

Figure 2.11 *Run/pass in lineball*

Thorpe) is convinced that the first game to play following the inclusion of the pass back rule is something like 4 *v* 1 (see Figure 2.12).

The rules of the game are as follows:

1. Attackers have 1 minute to score as many tries as possible.
2. Once a try is scored run back and start again.
3. If touched stop and pass. (Having a 'flag' (bib) tucked into the waist of the shorts, which must be removed to be counted as a touch, ensures no cheating and gives more chance to the runners.)
4. Offences like a dropped ball, interception, or ball thrown forward merely cause the team to return to the start line to begin again.
5. Defender starts on the half-way line until the first pass or run.

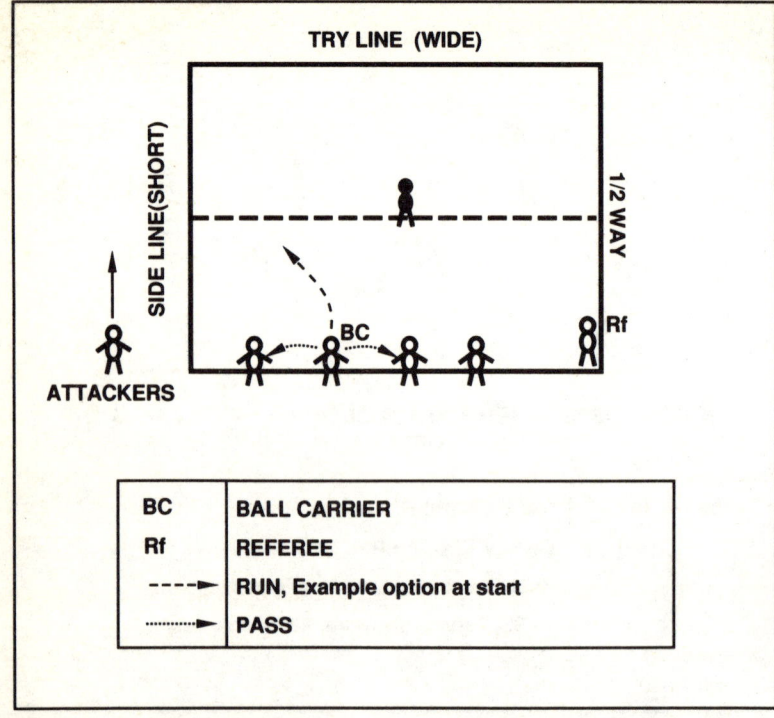

Figure 2.12   *4 v* 1 game including pass back

The decision to run or pass?
If the ball carrier stands still and passes what happens? The defender moves across and forward – the attackers have gone nowhere. If the ball carrier runs powerfully and takes on the defender what might happen? The attacker might beat the defender – the defender has to commit to stop the attacker, therefore other attackers are in space. The ball is in front of supporting players.

It is quite easy to make this into a little competition on a rotation basis. The defender works hard for one minute and carries the tries against him/her as the score. After one minute the defender becomes the referee (for a rest), the referee joins the attacking side, and one attacker becomes the defender. We feel that many children do not enjoy officiating because they only start when the game is complex, why not start when there are only one or two rules? In such a situation stress the following:

- the referee's decision is final;
- no arguing – you are wasting time; and
- defence is important in games.

The game encourages running skills, pace, swerve and scoring tries, passing develops in context.

By moving a few lessons forward the game may be 4 *v* 2 with a simple touch, hold, maul contact, ie now when the player is touched, (s)he must stop, turn and keep the ball available but they can push back toward the try line. The touching defender can embrace the attacker and resist the attackers push back. A simple controlled contact and maul is present.

The starting positions are exactly as in the first game but now there are two defenders. This can be a competition between three pairs. Each pair defending for two minutes against the other two pairs. (This is quite effective with three pairs of bibs, eg reds and blues take on yellows.)

The idea of an attacker running to make a defender commit him/herself to stopping the run (by touch or later a tackle) is obvious if you ask the question 'Do you think it is better to have four against two or three against one?' The answers vary.

Figure 2.13 indicates how committing one defender to the maul and then reacting to the position of the other, broadens the decision of whether to run or pass. Of course sometimes we have to go through two mauls to score but often the first defender committed to the maul is left behind, their defence has no depth.

As these elements are practised the sides can become more even but by then the children are becoming aware of the decisions to be made. To run or pass, to commit a player or open up the play, to go to the blind (closed) or open side. Concepts like depth in defence, pressuring the ball, making and using space are all here.

As the use of video material becomes available extracts from adult games can be shown. Forward drives on the blind side which set up runs for the three quarters will illustrate the points developed in the children's simpler game.

The decision about when to move on in the game is based largely on whether the children have grasped the concepts, they may never perfect the skills, that's why top players still play 4 *v* 2.

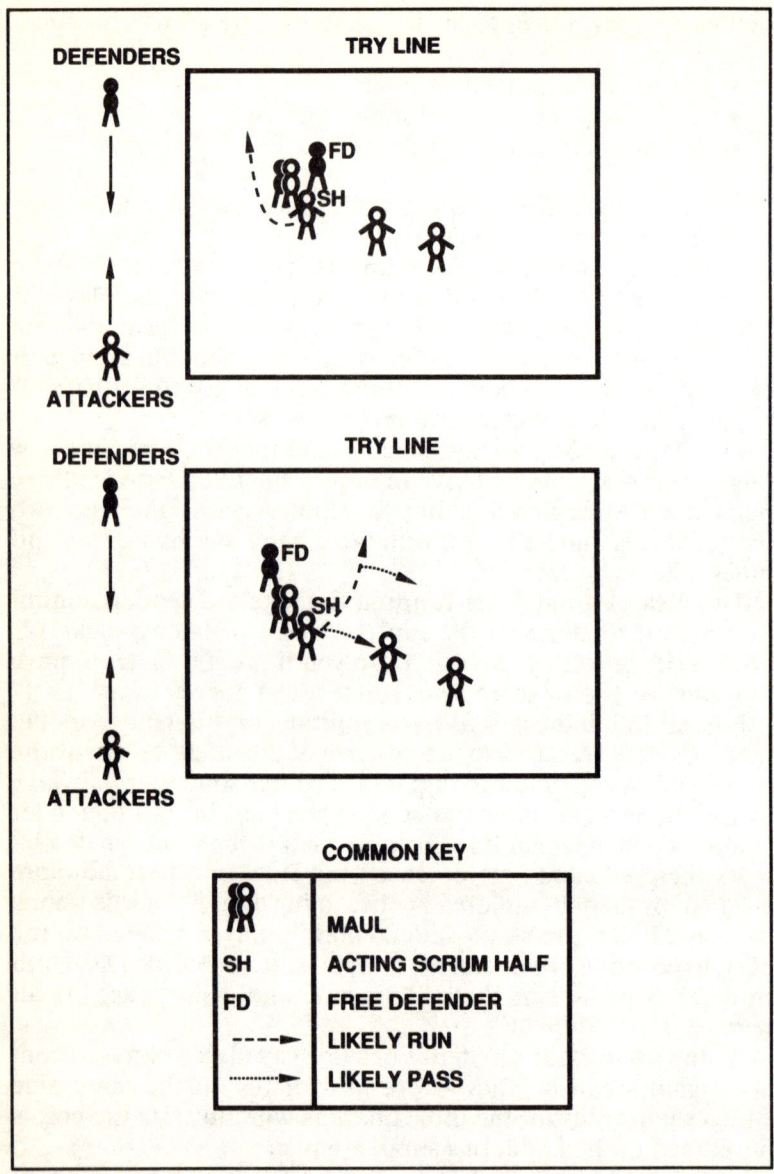

Figure 2.13 *Effect of changing position of defenders on running or passing*

A sports education

Once children understand the game in the sense that they appreciate the implications of the rules, have investigated the tactics involved, learnt to make appropriate decisions and answered problems as skilfully as they can, is their game development complete? We think not.

Let us suppose that the children have been taught the principles of divided court games, perhaps using throw catch games in the first year and then moved on to a form of badminton singles and doubles in the second and third years. Of course there is a need to practise and consider the finer tactical points but we would see also a need to broaden the knowledge investigated. Perhaps in the fourth and fifth years some of the focus should be on badminton in a fuller sense. As youngsters may now be using full courts for singles and doubles there will probably be times when some are sitting out. This seems the ideal time to begin some form of analysis. Our first attempt at this would be to suggest an analysis of the following points:

- How long (time) do the rallies last, how long is the rest between rallies (stop watch and record sheet). How many times do the players get the shuttlecock back in a five-minute spell (frequency table)?
- How many jumps in the air or sudden spurts (frequency table)?

This information can be followed by basic analysis, discussion and design of on-court drills and off-court training, thus the activity of a lesson might have a different balance, ie matchplay with analysis followed by high intensity exercise – pressure drills to ensure that the movement patterns identified are practised with overload.

This broadening of knowledge can move to consider the type of player who seems to be successful – perhaps light, fast, agile. A simple tabulation of which nationalities have players in the 'top 100' can lead to a discussion about the contributing effects of physique, culture or education. Equally, this broadening can fit well with the community link in that if badminton is a significant course, we see it as vital that the teacher helps children find out where they can play recreationally, play for a team, enter a competition or receive more coaching. This need not take away undue activity time and might well be co-ordinated within a GCSE course. We would expect some teachers to be using teaching styles in which children take some responsibility for their own and each other's learning, particularly as we feel sure that most skill practice will be at an individual level. With this background some simple observation of the biomechanics of a movement might be investigated, eg 'why' and 'how' the racket moves so fast. We have noted some interesting approaches to try and incorporate this form of input with an appropriate assessment for all children (see Chapter 9: Accreditation).

If a little time is spent in this area at the expense of hitting, but motivation is greatly enhanced to the extent that more children feel inclined to play outside the lesson and see sport as interesting, then this development is well worth while. What we must guard against most carefully with all the children, but particularly with the non-GCSE students, is that this becomes no more than an interesting academic exercise for the teacher.

The curriculum in the secondary school

It should now be apparent that if children are to understand the games they play and be fully involved in them both physically and mentally, then we must drastically rethink the way we teach games. Realistically we accept that it may take time to develop a 5–16 games education, but we feel that we have reached a point in our thinking about games that would allow us to propose a Secondary Games Programme which maintains the width necessary to reflect the different focus of games but gives sufficient depth to allow a game to be developed. It should be apparent that the length of time allocated to chosen games may differ. We believe that a person can be given a basic understanding of the game of badminton singles within eight to ten hours but might require perhaps 30 hours to reach a similar position in rugby football.

The programme is based upon the assumption that a specific game is developed along the following lines:

1. It grows out of the appropriate game in the foundation course – using and reinforcing the underlying principles inherent in that type of game.
2. The more specific concepts determined by the particular rules

of the specific game are investigated, with parallels made to related games.

3. The game is investigated in the wider context of physical and psychological demands, its place in the community/society. In taking this into account, a secondary programme might look as shown in Table 2.1 (see p 69).

Notes

a Any number of factors will have to be considered when sampling from invasion, court and fielding games.
b The sampled games will be continued in the third and fourth years.
c A decision might be taken to teach the same game in each of the three years, or the game might change from year to year.
d Court games do not require the same allocation of time as they are less complex tactically than the others.
e Courses in the fourth year are based upon sport education.

Conclusion

As we all know this is a time when fundamental changes are being made in the school curriculum. Most of us wait with bated breath for the publication of the national curriculum in which physical education is recognised as being one of the foundation subjects. From what we hear, it seems that curriculum time for PE might be cut by as much as half and a comment by Tom McNab in *The Times* (30 March 1988) that 'there is simply no hope of delivering skill with such a meagre allowance' is particularly relevant to the present discussion. We remain convinced that skill cannot be delivered given the present allocation of time let alone half of it, and that a major revision of our aims and objectives for games teaching is long overdue. Seen in this light, the current trend towards 'benchmarks' and 'behavioural objectives' could be a retrograde step, if we are not careful this will lead down the rocky road to 'tests and measurements' with teachers doing little more than taking a clipboard to the PE lesson.

This cannot be the way ahead. We do not view the games curriculum as a series of piecemeal experiences which somehow come together. The physical education teacher, in selecting a sample of games, must highlight the relationships between them and must develop them working with rule structures, increasing

YR	AUTUMN (14HRS)	SPRING (14 HRS)		SUMMER (10 HRS)
	FOUNDATION COURSE			
1.				
2.	INVASION [a] e.g. Basketball [b]	COURT [a] e.g. Badminton [b]	GAME [c] X	FIELDING [a] e.g. Cricket [b]
3.	INVASION	COURT [d]	GAME X_1	FIELDING
4.	INVASION [e]	COURT [e]	GAME X_2	FIELDING [e]
5.	NEW GAME e.g.Lacrosse	COMMUNITY LINKED COURSES		EXAMINATION TERM

Table 2.1 *A games curriculum: time allocation, one hour per week*

tactical complexity and greater decision-making capacity. It is the ability to think and operate in this way which separates the PE teacher from other providers of games experiences, eg coaches and sports leaders. Teachers should welcome the support of others, particularly with extra-curricular work, but a coherent 'Games Education' leading to a 'Sport Education', must be a major part of the *raison d'etre* of the PE teacher.

References

Bunker, D J and Thorpe, R D (1982) A model for the teaching of games in secondary schools. *Bulletin of Physical Education* 18, 1, 5–8.

Thorpe, R D, Bunker, D J and Almond, L (1986) *'Sport Pedagogy'. Proceedings of the Olympic Scientific Congress* Human Kinetics Publishers.

Chapter 3

Curriculum Developments in Gymnastics

Bob Smith

Introduction

At a seminar organised by HMI in Leeds during 1986 the results of an investigation into the state of gymnastics in schools were presented and revealed a very poor and depressing picture. Delegates discussed the erosion of time devoted to physical education in schools and the consequences for gymnastics which is an activity that needs time if real benefits are to be derived.

However, this is not the only problem, the diminishing time is only one reason for the decline in gymnastics in schools in recent years. This chapter attempts to identify some of the reasons for this decline before relating to the status quo and then turning to the future. One thing is becoming abundantly clear, if positive steps are not taken to improve and revitalise gymnastics in schools now, its future is very bleak and some feel that the expensive gymnasia equipment, used so frequently in the 1950s and '60s, will become merely a nostalgic relic.

The great divide in gymnastics

Following the vehement reaction against Swedish gymnastics, vaulting and agility and utilitarian military style physical training, the emergence of modern educational gymnastics was thought to be a new and exciting solution to the form gymnastics should take in schools. With child-centred education forming the backcloth of educational policy and manifesting itself in the publication of *Moving and Growing* in 1952, and *Planning the Programme* (1953) the stage was set for a new era.

Swedish physical training was regarded as outdated and of limited use, particularly as the new post-war focus of attention was on the child as an individual rather than children in general. The process of education was thought to be as important (some would say more important) as the product and gymnastics, like other aspects of physical education had to move with the times.

The original conception of modern educational gymnastics as proposed by Morisson (1956; 1960) placed the individual child at the centre of the phil-osophy. Work was to extend a child's tendency for natural movement while fostering the expression of individuality. However, in retrospect it is clear that somewhere along the line something has gone drastically wrong. The search for conceptual clarity of the early pioneers produced conceptual ambiguity and uncertainty on the part of many practitioners. The philosophy of modern educational gymnastics and the accompanying material appeared to be difficult to grasp for some teachers of physical education and much confusion reigned in the late 1950s and early 1960s as teachers emerged from training colleges and attempted to teach this new form of gymnastics. The cause of the confusion is difficult to pinpoint exactly but two issues have become clear.

The first pertains to the great divide between men and women's perceptions of gymnastics. Few men were able to follow in the footsteps of Laban favoured by women physical educators and in a characteristic response to the women's reactions to Swedish gymnastics, some men withdrew to a 'gymnastic skills' approach and became more resistant to change than ever. Men's and women's gymnastics became polar opposites with a 'never the twain shall meet' attitude. Some writers have portrayed this battle of the sexes in a light-hearted vein, and some amusing and often bizarre anecdotes have emerged. However, on a serious note, it would be wrong to dismiss the reaction of male physical educationists to educational gymnastics outright because some, notably Percy Jones (an advisor in Lancashire) in the 1960s, were very successful and very influential with a problem-solving approach that was not Laban based. Nevertheless, by the 1970s many men remained only marginally affected by developments in educational gymnastics. Some continued to teach vaulting and agility, some paid lip service to educational gymnastics with first- and second-year pupils and others lost their way altogether. Meanwhile, educational gymnastics was firmly established within women's physical education programmes in schools.

As time has progressed the material of gymnastics as perceived by men and women seems to have moved no closer together. As far as many men were concerned, Olympic gymnastics (sometimes referred to as artistic gymnastics) replaced the Swedish form, and vaulting and agility continued to dominate many men's perspectives in contrast to the so-called educational approach of the women. 'Educational' and 'Olympic' were bipolar opposites despite attempts in the men's training colleges to teach educational gymnastics with varying degrees of success; most of them were closer to Percy Jones' approach than the Laban-based approaches.

As we move into the 1980s a good deal of water has flowed under the bridge and in the light of the comments that have been made so far, it is now appropriate to look to the future, and to assess the role, scope and usefulness of gymnastics as a curriculum activity in the 1990s and beyond.

The 1960s and early 1970s proved to be the time of great polarization. The temporary boom in Olympic gymnastics in the 1970s, generated largely by Olga Korbut, did little to help schools' gymnastics in the long term, although it did seem to draw attention to the value of 'skills' once again. One of the misconceptions of some protagonists of modern educational gymnastics appears to have been that skills as such were not taught and yet the activity was perceived to be skilful (Morrison, 1960). This semantic dichotomy served to confuse and those opposed to modern educational gymnastics made a great deal of the lack of skills teaching. However, the true essence and value of 'educational gymanstics' is captured in the following quotation:

> In however transient and modest a way gymnastics, rightly conceived and taught, can be a means for the 'release of the individuality' of some of our pupils; we should at least hold to the ideal that we should be trying to make it happen for all our pupils. (Wright, 1982)

However, it is pertinent to note this quotation:

> Neither do men put new wine into old bottles. (Matthew, IX:17)

It is appropriate that the words of John Wright, a foremost authority in schools gymnastics over the past twenty years, should be cited at this stage in optimistic vein, tempered by the cautionary words of Matthew. For, there is always the possibility in a subject like gymnastics, that the same ideas are promoted under the pretext of a different slant or emphasis which would only be likely to be of short-term value.

Rethinking gymnastics

Often a refocus or reappraisal, however, is very necessary – so easy to say yet so difficult to achieve. There are many interested parties concerned with the state of gymnastics in schools in 1988, each with his or her own view, often strongly held, and no doubt based on sound reasoning and sound educational philosophy. However, for the first time in a long while there appears to be a degree of consensus emerging which would give credence to Wright's optimistic statement.

This consensus appears to be towards methodological and philosophical integration, 'the marriage of two ideologies living under one gymnastic roof' Smith (1986). The scope of this integration lies along a continuum which is broad enough to accommodate variations of style and approach but narrow enough to enable conceptual practicability (that is, to be readily understood and applied). The present writer's preference is towards the centre of the continuum for the most workable and useful form of gymnastics. But before considering these views it will be useful to consider John Wright's projections and those of Keith Russell in order that a fuller picture can be considered.

Wright has supported the teaching of educational gymnastics for well over twenty years but his teaching has been effective for at least three reasons. First, he acknowledges the importance of a high skill in his work, and is prepared to teach specific skills where necessary and appropriate. Second, he has the ability to motivate people to work at their skill threshold, that is, to their optimum potential, and third, he has a thorough understanding of the material of gymnastics and of the learning processes which underpin effective composition work.

In recognition of the perennial semantic problem with the prefix 'educational', he calls his work simply 'Gymnastics' and this title is to be strongly advocated as we move into the latter part of the 1980s. A crucial aspect of Wright's philosophy is that 'a freely variable gymnastic environment is widely exploited using apparatus in varied combinations and relationships', thus making it possible for children to experience a wide range of actions from the material of gymnastics. This environment also allows children the opportunity to extend their awareness and discrimination about the action potential of their bodies.

Skill according to Wright is manifested in three ways. First, mastering suitable selections from the action material of gymnastics – skilled body management. Second, creating individual phases of movement by the appropriate blending of whole body and part body actions and their spatial, dynamic and relationship variable features, and third, skill in the observation of movement by learning to look with increased awareness and discrimination at movement. This last point is particularly important if gymnastics is to have a real function in life. The cognitive aspect of kinaesthetic appreciation has endless possibilities in our culture where movement is central and essential. Another feature of gymnastics from Wright's perspective concerns the harnessing and fostering of individuality. As a supporter of child-centred educational philosophy, Wright stresses the importance of the child's creation of movement together with his personal pride in skilled body management and body awareness. This is closely linked with a clearly defined aesthetic focus in both the structuring and synthesis of movement in a qualitative form. This is a notion supported by many (myself included) but also by Garner (1985) who comments on the 'shape and line' of movements where 'the gymnast sets out and concentrates on the beauty, strength and flexibility of his movements', so that 'kinaesthetic satisfaction is gained by having got the skill/movement just right'.

Although Wright does not strictly adopt Laban's terminology in his teaching and his categorisation of the material of gymnastics, a point which differs from the early pioneers of the 'movement approach to educational gymnastics', he acknowledges his debt to some of Laban's insights. Such insights can form a helpful part of a teacher's knowledge so that he or she is better able to help children achieve a 'systematic exploration of open-ended tasks from which the new synthesis of phrase can arise' (Wright, 1975). Many would support this view but it should be pointed out that Laban's movement analysis is not universally acknowleged in gymnastics and some critical observers may regard it as positively inhibitory. The same criticism is sometimes made of the use of themes in gymnastics, even though they are used to provide order and systemisation to programmes.

Finally, underpinning the work proposed by Wright is a sound knowledge of principles: physiological principles as applied to the physical benefits of gymnastics; biomechanical principles as applied to movement analysis; principles of aesthetic design; and principles of safety, which in a world of increasing litigation is of paramount importance to the teacher of gymnastics. Most of all, he constantly emphasises the importance of his systematic classification of the action material of gymnastics which underpins all his planning, teaching and observation.

The quality of thinking in Wright's work is clearly evident but the cautionary note indicated by quoting Matthew's gospel earlier should be taken into account. Pupil centred gymnastics has been misinterpreted in the past and we must guard against it happening in the future.

The second projection for the future of gymnastics in schools comes from the Associate Professor of the University of Saskatchewan, Keith Russell. In 1985, the British Amateur Gymnastics Association (BAGA) Conference was devoted to 'Gymnastics in schools'. John Atkinson, the technical director, was very direct in his opening comments before giving Russell the floor.

> The straight fact is that educational gymnastics has not succeeded and that the BAGA has not really provided any answers which the PE Association of Great Britain and BAALPE could readily grasp. (Atkinson, 1985).

As far as the BAGA is concerned a new form of gymnastics must be sought and Russell has been asked to present an alternative to be 'weighed in the balance'.

Russell is quite explicit in his views and recognises his own rationalisation of the strength and weaknesses of the 'educational' and 'Olympic' styles of teaching in Britain. He appreciates the Laban inspired movement in education and how it encourages the teacher to understand the basic components of human movement, and he acknowledges the necessity of allowing individual exploration and discovery to 'explore for themselves the seemingly unlimited permutations, intricacies and nuances of human movement' (Russell, 1985).

However, as Russell poignantly points out, 'how long does one continue analysing movement?' One of the weakness of educational gymnastics he sees is that teachers are not trained to relate it to other forms of gymnastics or to gymnastics as a lifetime activity. Equally, he has misgivings about the Olympic approach on three counts. First, with so many skills to choose from, and with each curricula being different, it is an onerous task to produce a progressive programme. Second, the skills are often too difficult for children to perform in the school environment, and third, the Olympic style does not take account of individual differences.

His answer, therefore, is to provide an approach to gymnastics 'that represents a distillation or rarefaction of gymnastics into a few themes or movement patterns from whence most gymnastic skills evolve'. The distinction between the Laban-based themes and his themes is that the latter are derived from gymnastic origins (as are Wright's) and not borrowed from educational dance. He sees gymnastic skills as unique to gymnastics and upon this assumption he assembles his basic taxonomy in order to build a logical curriculum.

This utilitarian approach to human movement consists of six basic themes: landings, statics, swings, locomotions, rotation and spring which are explained clearly in a logical manner. With Laban's movement analysis superimposed upon them there appears to be a workable form of gymnastics which is specific, easy to understand, and which allows freedom for both teacher and child to explore their individuality. The child can create his own version or variation of a basic skill by simply altering the body parts used, the spatial dimensions used, the effort qualities used, or the relationship with others or with apparatus.

Russell sees this system of a sensible bridge between movement education and traditional gymnastics, as having a number of advantages:

1. It provides the basis for logical curriculum development.
2. It de-emphasises the restrictive nature of apparatus as specific skill learning.
3. It incorporates an awareness of safety, both in performance and understanding of performance.
4. It allows ample opportunity for exploration and creativity as well as individualised learning.

This far in the proceedings we have considered two projections for the future in an attempt to determine the way forward. However, the way forward will not be achieved in isolation as far as physical education, or indeed gymnastics, is concerned. As a historical perspective reveals, gymnastics has been modified in the light of general education developments, and it would be improper at this time not to take heed of comments made in recent publications concerning our schools.

The statements made in *The School Curriculum* (DES, 1981) provide the basis for 'the purposes of learning' and are re-emphasised in the White Paper – *Better Schools* in 1985. In the obvious vocational emphasis there is a comment on the purpose of learning which may be adopted by physical educationalists. The object is to:

> help pupils develop lively, enquiring minds, the ability to question and argue rationally and to apply themselves to tasks, and physical skills.

And the general aim is to produce a 'broad', 'balanced', 'relevant' and 'differentiated' curriculum.

Clearly, the noteworthy ingredients of the first statement are relevant in the teaching of gymnastics today. We must produce a system which requires that children think for themselves and respond rationally to movement situations and problems so that they can develop understanding and experience high quality movement. Equally the gymnastics curriculum we select must have some relevance in the lives of the children and, if possible, give them something that will be useful in post-school life.

In Coventry local education authority there is a major thrust in physical education to develop 'personal and social development' and while this has been criticised by some, as a 'bandwagon' clearly there is a place for social learning in gymnastics lessons and this should be encouraged whenever possible. Equally, teachers of gymnastics should take heed of the criticisms that we are over-directive and too interested in the production of skills learning (DES, 1985), and try to 'involve children in their own learning' (Belshaw, 1986).

These comments have implications for the way forward for gymnastics in schools on two major counts: first, regarding the content of gymnastics; and second in the use and adaptation of teaching styles. In view of this and other relevant facts the teaching of gymnastics in schools has been rationalised in my own work at Loughborough University.

In order to remove the ambiguity and uncertainty in the minds of students, sometimes as a result of teaching practice in schools, it has been necessary to omit misleading prefixes such as 'formal' which has negative, stereotype connotations, and 'modern educational' which implies that any other form is not educational and therefore inferior. Instead, the term 'Gymnastics for schools' is used.

This area should be an amalgam of both material and teaching method currently found at opposite ends of the gymnastic spectrum in order to provide greater width of challenge to children, and greater balance and relevance in any given school or community. The current practice of teaching one aspect of gymnastics in preference to another is narrow, restrictive and counter-productive. It is contrary to the needs of children which are clearly diverse. It is suggested, therefore, that a more realistic approach would be to utilise the material of so-called 'formal' gymnastics (where appropriate) with the more useful aspects of 'educational' work, and to embody a readily discernable area of work that allows for some degree of objectivity in terms of skill acquisition, along with the development of mobility, strength and local muscular endurance which might be harnessed to the creativity, aesthetic awareness and individual responsibility developed by open-ended problems traditionally featured in the teaching of 'educational' gymnastics.

Gymnastics in this context should provide a challenging experience in which a child can achieve some mastery over his body through the acquisition of skill. It can be helpful in establishing his identity in peer group situations and can allow him to become increasingly aware of his aptitudes and limitations. Through his experiences in the gymnasium a child can learn what it is to be faced by a challenge, learn to cope with success (and a lack of it), and learn to come to terms with fear (in a controlled way). Gymnastics can form the basis for learning about health-related exercise and provide opportunities for the child to learn something of the potential of gymnastics for enhancing the quality of their lives. Thus, gymnastics, can become important in and for their lives.

Gymnastics should demand that participants be alert, vital and capable of responding to the environmental forces which influence their actions. Activities selected should lead to skilful execution and the teacher should have a regard for both the product of the achievement and the process which leads to it. The intrinsic value of movement learning is as important as the end product. We should help children to build a repertoire of skills which can be modified, expanded and embellished according to needs.

Within this continuum there is scope for accommodating various teaching styles to open-ended work and at any point along the continuum the teacher may change styles according to the particular requirements of the moment. For example, an open-ended task may start the lesson implying an informal style where the teacher asks the children to provide the answers. However, if a common answer emerges, eg a cartwheel, the teacher can teach this skill directly in a formal manner. Equally, the children may be given the opportunity to teach each other in a reciprocal way thus involving themselves in the criteria of observation, assessment and correction and increasing their cognitive awareness, in the process. Mosston (1985) refers to these styles in his book *From Command to Discovery* where style A is direct teaching, style C reciprocal teaching and so on until style F is reached. Along the continuum from A to F the responsibility moves from the teacher to the learner so that gradually, and in the appropriate situations, the responsibility for learning is relinquished by the teacher and accepted by the pupil.

This notion of varying the style of teaching is a popular contemporary issue but one which is based on sound educational principles if used appropriately. By varying the method by which we present material to children we can stimulate them much more effectively and allow for individual responses which may offer creativity and a true sense of personal credibility.

In conclusion, there is some evidence that a consensus is developing as to the kind of approach required to improve the quality of gymnastics in schools in line with current educational philosophy and practice. I have cited my own philosophy against the backcloth of the work of John Wright and Keith Russell to show how common elements are emerging; the growth of a simple, effective and workable approach which is conceptually sound and possesses enough breadth to encompass diversity and hence greater relevance to a wide range of individual differences.

Gymnastics must be seen as a meaningful activity and it must be seen to be of benefit to the modern child. The physical gains in particular have, in my view, not been fully utilised in recent years and this may be an obvious attraction to the youth of today given the current interest in health issues. Let us hope that some resolve is met soon, that some consensus is achieved, and that gymnastics develops as it should in the future.

References

Atkinson, J (1985) *Gymnastics in Schools* BAGA Annual Conference, Birmingham.

Belshaw, P (1986) The changing face of physical education. *The Way Ahead*, BAALPE Conference, Loughborough.

Bilborough, A and Jones, P (1963) *Physical Education in the Primary School* University of London Press, London.

DES (1981) *The School Curriculum* HMSO, London.

DES (1985) *Better Schools* HMSO, London.

Garner, R (1985) A personal view of gymnastics in schools. *Bulletin of Physical Education* 21, 1:24.

Ministry of Education (1952) *Moving and Growing* HMSO, London.

Ministry of Education (1953) *Planning the Programme* HMSO, London.

Morison, R (1956) *Educational Gymnastics* Physical Education Association, London.

Morison, R (1960) *Educational Gymnastics for Secondary Schools* Physical Education Association, London.

Mosston, M (1985) *From Command to Discovery* Merrill, London.

Mosston, M and Ashworth, A (1986) *Teaching Physical Education* (3rd edn) Merrill, London.

Russell, K (1985) An alternative approach to school gymnastics. BAGA Conference.

Smith, R A (1986) Gymnastics in schools. The way forward. DES Conference, I M Marsh Campus, Liverpool.

Wright, J (1975) Gymnastics in the curriculum. *The Way Forward* Unpublished MA Dissertation, Nonington College.

Wright, J (1982) Presentation of an exciting and demanding gymnastics curriculum for all abilities. *Conference Papers*. I M Marsh Campus, Liverpool.

Chapter 4
An Integrated Approach to Swimming Development

Colin Hardy

Introduction

Swimming is an activity that attracts individuals from both sexes
and from all ages. The appeal is a many-sided one and is based
on one or more interrelated dimensions. These dimensions can
be divided into four distinguishable but often interrelated areas:
physical and physiological; psychological; social; and spiritual.

In the physical and physiological area the individual may talk
about 'feeling in shape', improving 'muscular strength and
endurance' and 'exercising weakened muscles'. With the psychological area some individuals 'feel exhilarated' and others feel
'more relaxed' after swimming. In many cases the swimming
pool becomes the social meeting place because of its 'all-the-
year' attraction and the low cost of entrance and equipment. The
feeling of 'becoming one' with nature is not uncommon in
swimming and some have found an 'inner satisfaction' from
moving freely in water (Hardy, 1987a).

In this chapter the pupil objectives for a swimming programme are outlined, followed by an explanation of how the
programme can be developed step by step to achieve these objectives. The example lesson plans show how the material can be
presented in the practical situation.

GENERAL PUPIL OBJECTIVES
What do we hope that pupils might gain from taking part in a
swimming programme?

1. They should become physically active individuals by getting
   involved in a variety of swimming programmes and showing
   control and versatility.

2. We should expect them to show a knowledge and understanding of swimming activities.
3. They should make responsible decisions in swimming situations and in programme preparation.
4. They should learn from, show care towards, and work with others in a swimming environment.
5. Personal meaning should be found through swimming activities.

It is hoped that by immersing pupils practically and mentally in swimming that they are able to get 'inside' the activity and find meanings that will encourage them to continue into later life. Also, it is hoped that pupils will develop and show responsible and caring attitudes in aquatic environments.

PREPARATION OF A SWIMMING PROGRAMME
How do teachers prepare a swimming programme in order to achieve these pupil objectives?
For teachers the process of preparing a swimming programme is developmental and can be divided into three distinct steps (Hardy, 1987b):

- learning to swim;
- development of swimming; and
- commitment to an aquatic environment.

During the first two steps the teacher must ask two questions:

1. What should the pupils be able to do?
2. What should the pupils know?

Step 1: learning to swim

There are three stages to this step of learning to swim. First, pupils must familiarise themselves with the water environment. Second, they must learn to orientate themselves in water and finally they must learn ways of controlled propulsion. In addition to the specific swimming concepts of familiarisation, orientation and controlled propulsion the more general concepts of safety, confidence and relaxation play an important part in this particular step.

FAMILIARISATION
What pupils should be able to do
On entering the water the pupil should be able to use the steps, slip into the water from the side and jump in.

On leaving the water the pupil should be able to use the steps and the side.

Walking while holding the side; walking singly, in pairs and in groups; walking in different directions; and walking backwards, forwards and sideways should be practised to ensure complete mobility.

To encourage mobility there are a number of game forms such as: circle and line games, use of balls, hoops and large buoyant equipment.

What pupils should know
The placement of clothing in the changing room, hygiene, and procedures for entering the pool should all be familiar.

Knowledge of the pool lay-out is essential, ie shallow and deep ends, toilets, working areas and the meaning of signs.

Pupils should know the pool regulations, ie expected behaviour, signals for entering and leaving the water and the emergency signal.

On leaving the pool the pupils should know how to exit from the pool, the dressing procedure and the location of the assembly point.

The pupils should possess the following swimming knowledge:

- the safest ways of entering and leaving the water;
- ways of moving safely in water; and
- ways of playing safely in water.

Teaching focus
The teacher should help pupils to:

- get involved in a swimming programme;
- gain a control of body and limb movements in entering and performing in shallow water;
- gain a knowledge and understanding of safety and hygiene procedures in swimming; and
- gain confidence in the swimming environment.

ORIENTATION
What pupils should be able to do

The pupil should be able to obtain the horizontal position and place the feet back on the bottom of the pool, glide with equipment, glide to and from poolside in prone, supine and side positions, and regain the feet effectively.

Control above and under the water is essential. The pupil should practise submerging and coming to the water surface with appropriate breath control, floating and treading water skills.

The pupil should be able to move through the water with and without support. With support, the pupil should find ways of using the arms and legs and move in different directions in different positions. Without support, the pupil can feel for the best 'hold' on the water and experiment to find the most effective propulsive movements.

What pupils should know

The basic facts related to buoyancy, such as Archimedes' principle, the density of the human body and of water.

Teaching focus

The teacher should help pupils to:

- gain a control of limb movements in various body positions on and below the water surface and in replacing the feet back on the bottom of the pool;
- gain a knowlege and understanding of the mechanical principles that act upon the floating body;
- become more confident and relaxed in the swimming environment.

CONTROLLED PROPULSION
What pupils should be able to do

The pupil should learn the breast stroke-type strokes, ie breast stroke, butterfly breast stroke, life-saving kick, 'Old English' back stroke, elementary back stroke and the inverted breast stroke.

This should be followed by the crawl-type strokes, ie front crawl, butterfly dolphin, back crawl and other strokes such as the side stroke and trudgeon.

Simple turns should be practised, for example spin turns for crawl-type strokes, pendulum turns for breast stroke-type strokes and 'other' strokes.

Dives should be practised, such as the plunge dive, the straight backswing and arms back start.

Kicking and pulling variations, using different equipment should also be tried.

What pupils should know
There should be a knowledge of propulsive movement, ie:

- pulling movements – the reasons for curved arm patterns and for high elbow techniques; and
- kicking movements – the reasons for extended feet and initiating movement from the hip in crawl-type kicks and the reasons for everted feet and circular leg action in breast stroke-type kicks.

They should also be familiar with the non-propulsive recovery movements and the reasons for fast, controlled techniques.

Knowledge of the most effective co-ordination of leg, arm and breathing movements for the different strokes contributes to improved stroke timing.

Understanding the significance of trajectory and entry improves diving technique.

Knowledge of form, wave and frictional drag helps the pupil to understand the principles of resistance.

Teaching focus
The teacher should help pupils to:

- gain a control of body and limb movements in the performance of various strokes, turns and dives in deep water; and
- gain a knowledge and understanding of the mechanical principles that act upon the body moving in water and in flight.

Step 2: development of swimming

This step is mainly concerned with the specific concept of watermanship with its recreational and competitive implications. Also, the general concepts of flexibility, strength and endurance become important in Step 2.

WATERMANSHIP

What pupils should be able to do

To achieve stroke improvement and turns the pupil should implement fitness programmes (Hardy 1988), perform a variety of schedules involving full stroke, pulling and kicking practices and spin, pendulum and tumble turns.

The pupil should be familiar with all aspects of safety, ie:

- life saving – resuscitation procedures, ability to tow and get someone from the water, use of equipment, awards;
- survival – ability to perform the skills of survival in deep water, awards; and
- situations, solving simulated problems.

Game forms such as water polo can be practised, learning the basic skills and making up a ball game in water, lead-up games, keeping to the rules of water polo, offensive and defensive strategies and officiating games.

Aesthetic aspects of watermanship can be practised such as:

- synchronised swimming – basic movements, routines, routines with music, rules for competition and officiating;
- diving – simple forward, backward, inward and twist dives, use of firm and spring boards, marking of dives and officiating.

What pupils should know

In training for fitness the pupil should understand training terms and the importance of flexibility, strength and endurance. The pupil should also know how to prepare a schedule.

Problem-solving skills should be learnt regarding life saving and survival. The pupil should understand the common principles that have to be applied in emergency situations.

The pupil should take part in competitive and recreational activities to understand the aesthetics of games and how movements are initiated. The pupil should know the appropriate rules of an activity and about team co-operation.

Teaching focus

The teacher should help pupils to:

- develop all-round swimming ability and show versatility in a variety of swimming situations;
- gain a knowledge and understanding of flexibility, strength and endurance in the improvement of performance;
- make decisions in swimming situations and in programme preparation; and
- co-operate and show a responsible and caring attitude in swimming situations.

PRESENTATION OF STEPS 1 AND 2

As these two steps are so important in developing an intrinsic interest in the aquatic area, the teaching styles used must be flexible and allow for the many individual differences (Mosston and Ashworth, 1986). However, the approach actually used will depend upon the goals and setting for the teaching-learning event, the multiple perspective brought to the event by the teacher and pupils and what is expected from the event. For example, in trying to perform a dive early on in the programme a command style may be used because the pupils are inexperienced and the teacher may be concerned about safety. However, the performance of a synchronised swimming routine, at a later stage in the programme, may need a more inventive approach. Such a situation often invites skilled pupils to discover different solutions to a problem and the teacher may feel that a divergent style is the best way of achieving this.

By using a variety of styles and, where possible, involving the pupils in the planning and decision-making processes, it is hoped that pupils' initial interest will blossom into a meaningful commitment to the activity.

EXAMPLES OF LESSON DEVELOPMENT IN STEPS 1 AND 2

These lessons are only examples of how the work can be put into practice, and they are not intended as detailed lesson plans. An integrated conceptual approach is essential in Steps 1 and 2 as meanings can only be found by doing and understanding. The 'teaching focus' helps the teacher to see the overall perspective and the 'lesson instructional objectives' are to challenge the pupils. However, it must be noted that at any stage in a pupil's swimming development past ideas and practices are continually interrelated with new ideas and practices, and progress is made on both the physical and mental fronts, depending upon the development levels of the pupils.

Table 4.1 *Example lesson 1*

Situation	Activity	Question/teaching point	Teaching checks
Changing rooms	Change quickly	Have you placed your clothes tidily?	Check for clean feet and knees
	Go through the showers	Did you shower properly?	
Pool surrounds	Walk to the shallow end of the pool with your partner	Did you stay close to your partner?	Check for any pupil running or slipping
Shallow end of the pool	Walk down the steps holding on to the side of the pool		
	Walk in different directions holding on to the side of the pool	Slide the feet along the bottom of the pool	Check that pupils are working in pairs
	Walk holding your partner's hand and staying close to the poolside	Do you feel balanced when you walk in water?	Are the pupils in control of their body movements in shallow water?
	Walk in shallow water in all directions staying close to your partner		
Shallow end of the pool	Throw a ball to your partner	Can you keep the ball off the water surface?	Are the pupils still in control during the game forms?
	Make up a game for two	Did you keep to the rules?	
Shallow end of the pool	Walk as many widths as possible staying close to your partner	Can you use your arms for balance?	How many pupils achieved the objectives?

Example Lesson 1

FAMILIARISATION
The teaching focus could cover:

- correct safety and hygiene procedures; and
- control of the body and limb movements on entering the pool and while in contact with the bottom of the pool.

The instructional objectives of the lesson are:

- carry out the changing room procedures correctly and walk to the shallow end of the pool;
- enter the shallow end of the pool without help;
- play with a ball in the shallow end of the pool; and
- walk a minimum of four widths without making contact with the side of the pool.

The activities and objectives of this lesson are shown in Table 4.1.

Example lesson 2

FAMILIARISATION
The teaching focus could cover:

- correct safety and hygiene procedures; and
- control of the body and limb movements in a variety of pool entries and game forms.

The instructional objectives of the lesson are:

- carry out the established procedures before entering the shallow end of the pool;
- enter the shallow end of the pool in three different ways;
- play with your partner using a piece of equipment (ie ball, hoops); and
- play in fours using another piece of equipment.

The activities and objectives of this lesson are shown in Table 4.2.

Table 4.2 *Example lesson 2*

Situation	Activity	Question/teaching point	Teaching checks
Changing rooms	Go through the pre-swimming routines	Did you carry out the routine?	Are you satisfied that the pupils have established the routines?
Poolside and shallow end of the pool	Practise three ways of getting into the pool	Can you find different ways of walking down the steps?	Can the pupils enter the water safely?
	Get out of the pool using the steps	Can you find different ways of getting in from the poolside?	Make sure that pupils are getting in and out of the pool safely
Anywhere in the shallow end of the pool	Select a piece of equipment and play with your partner	Find different ways of using the piece of equipment. Can you play with the piece of equipment out of, on and under the water?	Are the pupils growing in confidence?
Anywhere in the shallow end of the pool	Select a new piece of equipment and play with your partner and two others	Can you do different things with this piece of equipment?	Are the pupils playing together safely?

Example lesson 3

ORIENTATION
The teaching focus could cover:

- control of the body in various floating positions and in placing the feet back on the bottom of the pool; and
- movement through the water using a variety of limb movements and body positions with the help of an aid.

The instructional objectives of the lesson are:

- select an aid and support the body in vertical, prone and supine positions;
- propel the body forwards in any position using arm and leg movements while supported by an aid;
- 'swim' a minimum of four widths while supported by an aid; and
- replace the feet on the bottom of the pool from prone and supine positions while supported by an aid.

The activities and objectives of this lesson are shown in Table 4.3.

Example lesson 4

ORIENTATION
The teaching focus could cover:

- control of the body and limb movements while in the horizontal position; and
- feeling the 'support' of the water.

The instructional objectives of the lesson are:

- glide to the poolside;
- glide away from the poolside in the prone and supine positions;
- glide away from the poolside in the prone and supine positions and replace the feet on the bottom of the pool; and
- 'swim' at least five metres with any combination of limb movements.

The activities and objectives of this lesson are shown in Table 4.4.

Table 4.3 *Example lesson 3*

Situation	Activity	Question/teaching point	Teaching checks
Changing rooms	Go through the pre-swimming routines	Are you all aware of the importance of these procedures?	Ask questions about hygiene
Poolside and then anywhere in the shallow end of the pool	Select an aid and support the body	Can you keep your feet off the bottom of the pool?	Comment on the lift (or upthrust) that the pupils appear to get in the water
	Support the body in various positions	Can you support your body in upright, back and front positions?	
	Try and move while supported	Can you move forwards, backwards, diagonally and in a circle?	
Shallow end and to one side of the pool	Swim a minimum of four widths while supported by an aid	What arm and leg movements did you use? Did you change your position and arm movements?	Check that the pupils are adjusting to the more horizontal position
Anywhere in the shallow end of the pool	Practise getting in the horizontal position and getting the feet back on the bottom of the pool	Did you get your head up? Did you tuck up? What did you do with the arms?	Check whether the pupils had any difficulty getting their feet back on the bottom of the pool because of the upthrust

Table 4.4 *Example lesson 4*

Situation	Activity	Question/teaching point	Teaching checks
Changing rooms	Go through the pre-swimming routines		Ask questions about safety
Close to the poolside and in the shallow end of the pool	Practise pushing and gliding to the poolside	Keep the shoulders under the water surface	Check whether the pupils are moving into the horizontal position easily
	Practise pushing and gliding away from the poolside and regaining the feet	Can you get your legs close to the water surface?	
Close to the poolside and in the shallow end of the pool	Practise gliding, and pulling and kicking to the poolside	Did you get into a horizontal position before touching the poolside?	Are the pupils in control in the horizontal position?
	Practise gliding, and pulling and kicking away from the poolside		
Anywhere in the shallow end of the pool	Holding a float practise gliding and kicking across the pool	Were you kicking with the body in the horizontal position?	Do the pupils realise they can maintain the horizontal position with a minimal amount of kicking?
Shallow end and to one side of the pool	Push and glide away from the poolside and see how far you can swim	Did you manage 5 metres?	Check for controlled arm and leg movements

Example lesson 5

CONTROLLED PROPULSION
The teaching focus could cover:

- effective arm propulsive patterns; and
- knowledge and understanding of arm propulsive patterns.

The instructional objectives of the lesson are to:

- swim 25 metres on a crawl-type stroke in deep water;
- swim 25 metres on a breast stroke-type stroke in deep water; and
- answer correctly one question on the pulling action used in the swimming strokes.

The activities and objectives of this lesson are shown in Table 4.5.

Example lesson 6

CONTROLLED PROPULSION
The teaching focus could cover:

- efficient stroke recoveries; and
- knowledge and understanding of streamlining.

The instructional objectives of the lesson should be:

- swim 25 metres breast stroke demonstrating a streamlined recovery action;
- swim 25 metres back crawl demonstrating a streamlined recovery action; and
- dive and glide a minimum of five metres.

The activities and objectives of this lesson are shown in Table 4.6.

Table 4.5 *Example lesson 5*

Situation	Activity	Question/teaching point	Teaching checks
Deep end of the pool	Swim widths on a variety of strokes	How many different strokes did you do? How did you pull your hand back?	Emphasise the curved movement of all pulling actions
Deep end of the pool	Swim widths on a crawl-type stroke	Can you feel the curved pulling action?	Explain the importance of finding 'still' water
Deep end of the pool	Swim widths on a breast stroke-type stroke	Can you still feel the curved pulling pattern? Why is the curved pulling pattern important?	Explain that the curve can be in the horizontal and vertical planes
Deep end of the pool	Swim widths on pulling practices alternating breast stroke and front crawl arm actions each width	Keep the elbows up	Emphasise this teaching point as it is basic to a correct pulling action
Deep and shallow ends of the pool	Swim one length on a crawl-type stroke	Did you keep the elbows up?	
	Swim one length on a breast stroke-type stroke	Why do you pull in a curved pattern?	
Shallow end of the pool	Teacher briefly summarises the arm propulsive pattern	When do you find you get a better 'hold' of the water? When do you find you 'slip' the water?	

Table 4.6 *Example lesson 6*

Situation	Activity	Question/teaching point	Teaching checks
Deep end of the pool	Practise pushing and gliding from the poolside in various body positions	What did you find was the most efficient body position?	Emphasise the importance of the near-horizontal position for swimming
	Practise pushing and gliding from the poolside with the limbs in various positions	What did you do with the arms and legs to maintain a fast glide?	Explain the importance of keeping the arms and legs straight and in line with the body
Deep end of the pool	Swim widths on breast stroke	Did you recover the arms quickly? How did you recover the arms? Did you stretch the arms forwards?	Check that the arms are moved inwards and forwards in a continuous movement
Deep end of the pool	Swim widths on back crawl	Did you recover the arms high?	Emphasise that the vertical recovery prevents any sideways body deviation
Stand on the poolside at the deep end	Practise diving and gliding in a streamlined position for distance	Did you stretch from the fingertips to the toes?	Emphasise the 'narrowness' of the gliding position
Deep and shallow ends of the pool	Dive into the deep end and swim one length breast stroke	Did you recover the arms within or close to the body limits?	Check that all arm recoveries help with the streamlining of the body
	Push and glide from the shallow end and swim one length back crawl		

Example lesson 7

WATERMANSHIP
The teaching focus could cover:

- showing versatility in several swimming situations; and
- reasons for using specific tows.

The instructional objectives of the lesson are:

- tow a supported subject 10 metres using a chin tow with a non-rigid aid;
- swim for five minutes without touching the poolside; and
- swim 50 metres using a life-saving kick.

The activities and objectives of this lesson are shown in Table 4.7.

Example lesson 8

WATERMANSHIP

The teaching focus could cover:

- selection of a schedule appropriate to swimming ability;
- self-control in completing a swimming schedule; and
- evaluation of the work.

The instructional objectives of the lesson are:

- complete the swimming schedule in less than 30 minutes;
- note the problems encountered in performing the schedule; and
- evaluate the schedule and discuss future schedules with the teacher and peer group.

The activities and objectives of this lesson are shown in Table 4.8.

Step 3: commitment to an aquatic environment

A commitment by pupils to continue involving themselves in an aquatic environment is dependent on many factors:

Table 4.7 *Example lesson 7*

Situation	Activity	Question/teaching point	Teaching checks
Deep end of the pool	Swim widths using different backstrokes	How many different strokes can you do?	Are the pupils using different types of limb movements?
	Swim widths using a life-saving kick	Circle the legs	
Deep end of the pool	Partner to float horizontally with a supporting aid between the legs: tow the partner for two widths using a life-saving kick and a chin tow	Did you keep your kick below your partner's body?	Do the pupils know when to use a chin tow?
	Partners change		
	Repeat practices several times		
Deep end of the pool	Partner to float horizontally with a supporting aid between the legs; tow the partner for two widths using a non-rigid aid	Did you keep your distance from your partner?	Do the pupils know when to use a non-rigid tow?

	Partners change position	
	Repeat practices several times	
Deep end of the pool	Swim for five minutes continuously in a clockwise direction without touching the poolside	Did the pupils adapt their strokes for continuous swimming?
Deep end of the pool	Circle the legs	
	Swim 50 metres in widths on a life-saving kick	Check that the leg kicks are becoming effective life-saving actions

Table 4.8 *Example lesson 8*

Situation	Activity	Question/teaching point	Teaching checks
Poolside	Check that the practices are understood	Have you decided on a clockwise or anti-clockwise direction?	Are you satisfied that the pupils have selected appropriate schedules?
	Organise all the equipment on the poolside in the shallow end	Have you checked the direction with the other lane swimmers?	
Start in the shallow end of the pool	Go through the schedule	Did you find any easy or difficult practices?	Are the pupils acting responsibly?
Shallow end of the pool	Discuss any problems encountered with the teacher and peer group	Did you finish all practices with good technique?	Do the pupils have a good understanding of how to perform the practices?
	Evaluate the schedule performance and indicate future developments	Did you follow the speed levels indicated for each practice?	Check the pupils' evaluation procedures

- the interest that the teacher has 'sparked off' in Steps 1 and 2;
- the opportunities that are offered at school and in the local community;
- the accessibility and cost of the available resources;
- the help given to the development of known activities or the learning of new aquatic activities; and
- social pressures, particularly those of the peer group.

This commitment to an aquatic environment can be developed in three ways. First, pupils may join a local life-saving or competitive swimming club to try to improve their present skills. Second, the pupils may want to use their swimming skills in learning a new activity such as sub-aqua diving. Third, the confidence gained from their swimming programme may motivate them to take up such sports as rowing, canoeing, wind-surfing and sailing.

Teaching Focus
Encourage pupils to assess their development and ascertain the value of the work.

Summary

The author has presented a way of integrating the theory and practice of swimming in the physical education curriculum, and Figure 4.1 illustrates how pupil objectives, swimming concepts and the teaching focus are interrelated.

References

Hardy, C A (1987a) The case for swimming, *British Journal of Physical Education*, **18**: 4, 187–9.

Hardy, C A (1987b) A model for learning to swim. *Swim*, Spring, 4–7.

Hardy, C A (1989) *Swimming for Fitness – A Progressive Programme*. The Health and Physical Education Project, Loughborough University of Technology. Publishers to be announced.

Mosston, M and Ashworth, A (1986). *Teaching Physical Education* (3rd Ed.). Merrill Publishing Co, London.

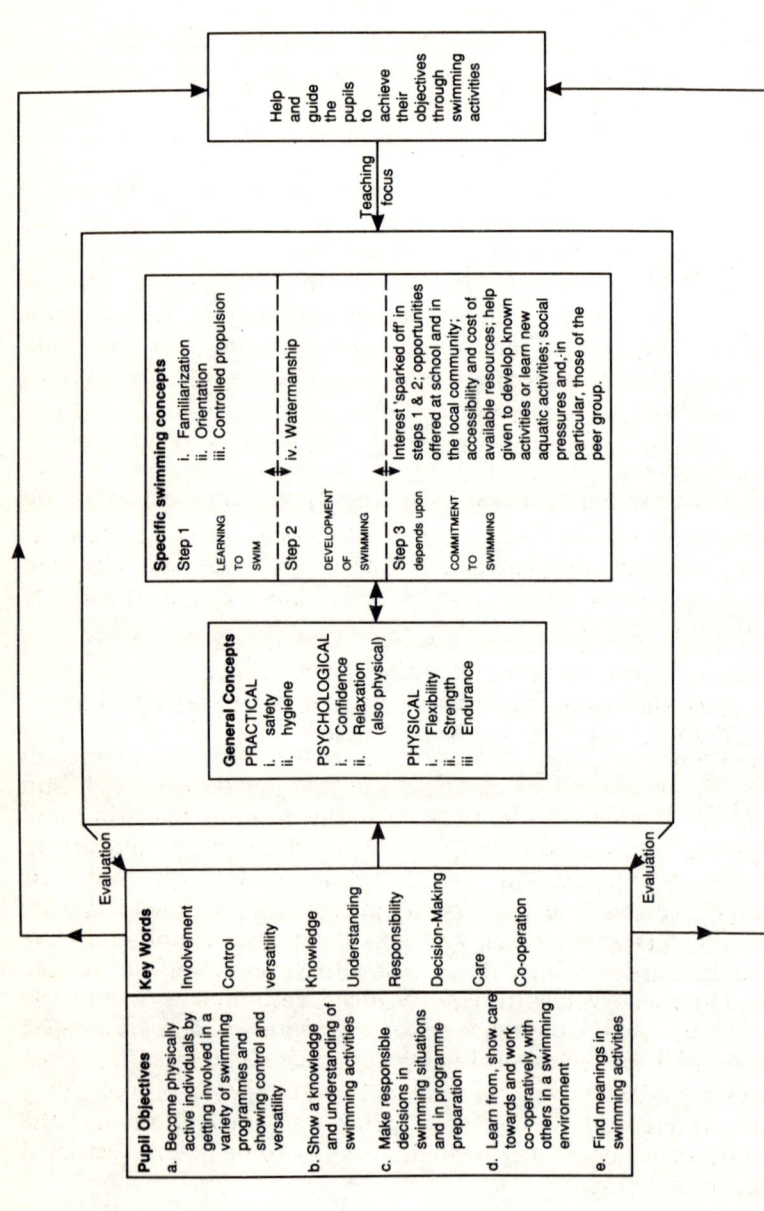

Figure 4.1 *The interrelationship between pupil objectives, swimming concepts and teaching focus*

Chapter 5

Reconstructing a Different Perspective for Athletics

Len Almond

Introduction

In this chapter I would like to propose a framework for establishing athletics within the physical education programme, especially in primary schools and the middle years of schooling, which could have a significant impact in the later secondary years. In order to stimulate debate and challenge existing thinking about the role of athletics in schools, I shall construct a theoretical position about athletics which has been used as a guideline to try out ideas in primary schools, secondary schools, and with students in higher education. Thus, the position that I shall take has been disciplined by practice in schools which has informed the nature of the framework.

Constructing a framework to develop athletics

The framework is based on the idea that from the fundamental movement patterns of children, the raw material of track and field athletics can be identified. Walking, running, throwing, and jumping have always been recognised as basic movement patterns (Gallahue, 1982) which provide us with our basic raw material. From these movement patterns it is possible to identify specific challenges which have stood the test of time and have resulted in their selection as competitive events for festivals like the Olympic Games or the World Championships, and the numerous national and local competitions, which have been formalised into competitive structures. These competitive structures have been taken as models for athletics in schools; they have influenced the physical education curriculum and the nature of what has been taught, and to some extent restricted their development.

However, it is possible to start with the basic raw material and construct an alternative framework for experiencing athletics in schools. Instead of moving from the raw material of athletics into formal events, I propose that teachers examine their action possibilities which opens up a whole host of new and different challenges. I am sure that it may be possible to conceptualise and reconstruct such action possibilities in a number of different ways, but I would like to propose a simple heuristic to take the initiative and present a potential framework. Figure 5.1 repre-

Material of athletics	Action possibilities
Walking	Acceleration over a short distance Endurance activities where pacing is important

Running	Acceleration over a short distance
	Endurance activities where pacing is important
	• with obstacles/barriers (high or long):
	  (a) constant or irregular distance between barriers
	  (b) constant or irregular height of barrier
	• on different terrain and surfaces:
	  (a) flat
	  (b) hills
	  (c) uneven surfaces (field/woodland)
	• with partners or individual

Jumping	Hopping, Leaping, and Springing
	• (a) high
	  (b) long (single, multiple, combination)
	  (c) assisted (eg pole) high or long
	• (a) standing or
	  (b) with a run

Throwing	Pulling, pushing, slinging
	• (a) height
	  (b) distance
	  (c) at targets
	• (a) sitting
	  (b) standing
	  (c) running

Figure 5.1 *A classification of action possibilities for athletics*

sents a classification of action possibilities which outlines a potential range of challenges to broaden the athletic experience of all young people. In this framework I see the action possibilities as the basis for recognising three distinct phases of the athletic experience.

Phase 1   Integrated play
Phase 2   The athletic form
Phase 3   Athletics as a sport

These phases provide an opportunity for introducing young people to the whole range of athletic experiences and challenges leading to the opportunity of competing with others, the appreciation of athletic endeavours and the spectacle of an athletic event. As a result there is the possibility that athletics could become an activity that one chooses to pursue because of its inherent satisfactions and become an important part of one's lifestyle.

The integrated play element

In the first phase of the framework I believe it is important that young children in the early primary years should be exposed to athletic challenges emerging from the basic raw material of movement. The action possibilities of walking, running, jumping and throwing can be used as a basis for integrating the play element within children's movement education. Thus, running and throwing are part of games experiences, and jumping can be seen as a component of dance and expressive movement and also in gymnastic movement themes. It is possible to construct a whole range of athletic challenges within the integration of play and movement experiences. The major difficulty is to ensure that in the planning process it is possible to achieve coherence as one integrates the action possibilities of athletics with the requirements of games, expressive movement, or gymnastic type activities. At the same time the skilful teacher has to consider how the whole movement experience can emphasise the joy of being active and the arousal of positive feelings associated with such participation.

The athletic form

Emerging from the integrated play element is a more definite focus which I call the athletic form. In Figure 5.2 the athletic form has three clear dimensions.

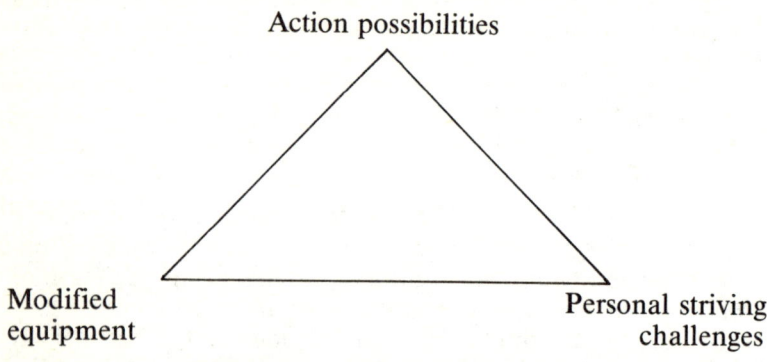

Figure 5.2 *The athletic form*

The first dimension, the action possibilities, provides guidelines for making a selection of challenges and sampling the potential of athletics. These challenges provide opportunities for testing oneself and striving to improve on one's best. Thus, in the second dimension, personal striving is concerned with attempting to achieve personal targets with an emphasis on the satisfaction to be gained from doing one's best. This is an important point because athletics is often seen as a competition with others in which striving to win is the challenge. In this chapter I would like to make a clear distinction between personal striving and striving to win because the former is a central feature of Phase 2 whereas the latter is central to Phase 3.

In athletics young people are usually asked to run against others over a set distance, eg 80 metres, and at the end a rank order of competitors is produced as a result of the participants striving to outrun their opponents. There is nothing wrong with this so long as it is acknowledged as only one way of indicating success and it is recognised that for some young people such a situation is a negative experience. Those young people who are obese, or frail, or those who are a long way behind their more mature peers, or whose body clock runs more slowly will repeatedly recognise that they are no good at this activity if they continually come last in a race and a long way behind their peers. There is little likelihood that they will derive satisfaction from this experience. Every time they are asked to compare themselves against others this message is reinforced and they learn that athletics is not for them. Some people would argue that they will find a niche in some other more appropriate activity, but this ignores an important point. If we accept this, we deny young people the opportunity for further development and reinforce the view that rewards are not for effort and determination, but for maturity. As teachers we need to help young people to identify physical education as a good experience and one in which they can try to do their best.

I would argue, therefore, that there is a need to shift the current focus within athletics and recognise that there is a prior concern to an emphasis on striving to win. Personal striving is important as a first priority because it has a different focus in which pupils have the opportunity to achieve satisfaction from their performance and to monitor their achievements. The challenges in Phase 2 provide opportunities for all pupils to experience success from their efforts and recognise improvements in performance. One example will serve to illustrate this. A class can be divided into pairs, one running and one assisting with recording achievement, and set the challenge of seeing how far they can run in four seconds. Their achievement is recorded by their partner. The runner is asked to try three times to see if they can surpass their first achievement, then they change places with their partner. Each pupil will usually exceed their first efforts or at least be very close. The shift in focus ensures that pupils are striving against their own efforts and social comparison is not used to indicate success. Some critics may retort that young people will automatically compare what they have done with others. Of course, some pupils will do this, but time after time when I have demonstrated this, observers have noted that pupils are centrally concerned with their own performance and satisfaction comes from their own efforts. Many more of these challenges have been identified in a booklet produced by the Health Education Authority Project, Health and Physical Education based at Loughborough University (Almond, 1988).

In the third dimension it is necessary to modify equipment, especially for hurdling and throwing challenges in order that the technical limitations imposed by inappropriate equipment, eg heavy shots and a large discus, are reduced. Thus, in hurdling the type of barriers, the height, and the distances between each barrier can be modified. Too often young people have to adjust to the inappropriate demands of the event rather than modify the event to enable a person to perform adequately. Hurdling is about the rhythm of moving fast over a specified distance with obstacles which have set distances between them. Thus, if we start off with the idea of three strides and striding over an obstacle, we can teach young people the rhythm of hurdling, and increase the distance between obstacles and their height as they become more competent and acquire the confidence to run fast over a barrier. In throwing, a whole range of new objects can be introduced, eg quoits or hoops for slinging actions; netballs/footballs/ volleyballs for heaving, pushing and slinging; old worn-out rounders bats or rhythmic gymnastic clubs for pulling actions; old woollen socks filled with sand or blasting shot for pushing, pulling, or slinging. The important point is not to be restricted by current conceptions of what constitutes adult throwing implements.

During this phase it is unnecessary to emphasise the technical aspects of performance, but it is important to ensure that challenges are underpinned by the use of key teaching cues or principles of action, eg in throwing think of 'long and tall'. At this stage key words become part of a pupil's vocabulary which they can incorporate into their performances. The challenges that teachers present need to be underpinned by key biomechanical principles in order that key root movements can become part of the pupil's experiences of athletics. Therefore the kind of challenge that is presented, the key words used to reinforce it, and teacher interventions provide the means for developing major root movements.

Athletics as a sport

The dominant focus in Phase 2 was the idea that athletic challenges should have a personal context in which all pupils can recognise that athletics can be personally rewarding and that achievement can be a product of their own efforts. From this phase of the athletic form, the third phase emerges as 'athletics as a sport'. After Phase 2 many young people will wish to test themselves against others in structured competitive situations. In such a context teachers and coaches will wish to provide opportunities to compete appropriate to pupils' developing physical needs, and mindful of long term developments. Thus, young people can learn how to compete, how to enjoy the struggle of a 'good' competition, and recognise that thorough preparation is part of producing one's best and stretching one's capabilities. In addition they can learn to respect other competitors and see them not as obstacles to their own success but as contributors to a 'good' contest.

Phase 3 which can be seen in Figure 5.3 contains three major components:

1. Recognised competitive events
2. Standard equipment
3. Striving to win: challenges

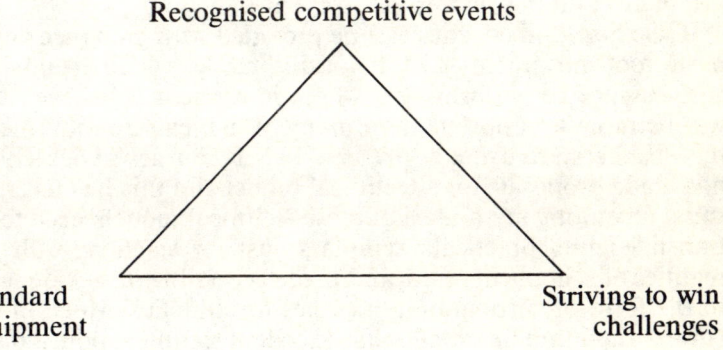

Recognised competitive events

Standard equipment

Striving to win challenges

Figure 5.3 *Athletics as a sport*

The action possibilities of Phase 2 become more formalised so that competition can take place within a clearly defined range of events. The equipment required for these events may have to be modified in order to reduce any technical limitations, but there is a clear emphasis on standard distances, implements, and regulations governing conduct so that a structure for competition against others can take place. As a sport the challenges within Phase 3 are based on striving to win where one attempts to excel worthy opponents. Here the challenge is clearly one in which rank orders are established and participants are aware of this point and still wish to compete.

During Phase 3 athletes will wish to practise in order to enhance their performances. Thus, at this stage the idea of a basic working model, arising from the root movement patterns of Phase 2, is introduced to enable performers to execute movement patterns effectively and with maximum efficiency. But, such a working model needs to be seen as a whole movement and not a scaled down version of adult performers. A basic working model is a representation of mature movement and not simply a mini-version. This idea is important for young people because there is a danger that the technical requirements of an event will be broken down and specific features rehearsed over and over again. Also, there is the danger that some techniques adopted by young athletes, even though they appear effective, are dead-end models which lead the athlete down a path that may be impossible to change and may impair future improvements. There is a need to provide basic working models that incorporate the technical demands of an event, appropriate biomechanical principles and the rhythm of an event in action.

If teachers and coaches can be provided with guidance about basic root movements and a working model which retains the very essence of performing a whole movement, I believe these will be more appropriate than many of the lead-up movements that teachers are using at present. This is not new, Dick (1986) has made proposals for a technical model and this has taken us some way along my route, but these technical models need to be translated into practical exemplars, just for teachers, with the realities of schools in mind, and made accessible on a wide scale in the form of curriculum guidelines for athletics. Much of the current literature in athletics has excellent technical points but it rarely tackles the problem of how young people can grasp athletics in its simplest form within a school physical education pro-gramme.

Alternative uses for athletics

We must not assume that the only potential use of school athletics is the preparation for competitive situations. Some young people, after their involvement in Phase 2, may not choose to enter into competitions against others and yet they may wish to continue with athletics. We should respect this right and consider what provision we could make to maintain their interest and commitment. Some young people will continue to enjoy being challenged in an athletic context, for others they may wish to choose running for their health or simply enjoy the satisfaction of being active. It may be that athletic challenges in unusual forms could be part of a festival of activity in which teams compete for recognition or acclaim within the school or between schools. The television programme 'It's a Knockout' provided the inspiration for constructing a festival which stimulates and awakens interest in athletic challenges which are more open ended and exhilarating.

Such a festival would require preparation in the form of conditioning, planning, and identifying appropriate challenges which simulate what they might expect on the day.

In the same way, school sports days and athletics meetings could be injected with more imagination and originality to enable large groups to participate, using a range of alternative athletic challenges – including competition against others – so that the whole school could obtain real value from the occasion. Instead of repeating the same type of sports day each year, examine alternatives which involve the whole school, or a year group, and generate excitement, commitment, and the satisfactions of enjoying athletics. If your sports day does this – fine – but check this out by undertaking an inquiry to find out what pupils, staff, and parents actually feel about the day and preparation for the day.

Conclusion

In conclusion, I would like to summarise what I am proposing. First, I am suggesting that athletics should not be dominated by traditional adult stereotype events, but should be based on the action possibilities that arise from the raw material of athletic movement. These action possibilities provide a framework for reconstructing athletics in order to explore their potential as athletic challenges in a physical education programme. Such a reconstruction should involve three phases which provide a lead into athletics as a competitive sporting activity and provide the means by which young people can either choose to opt into a competitive situation against others or continue with athletics as an opportunity for personal striving. Underpinning an individual's performance is the need to learn root movements and a basic working model to enhance their achievement.

References

Almond, L (1989) *A Health Focus in Athletics* To be announced.
Dick, F (1986) *But First . . .* British Amateur Athletic Board, London.
Gallahue, D L (1982) *Understanding Motor Development in Children*, John Wiley & Sons, Inc, New York.

Chapter 6

Developments in Outdoor Education and Residential Experience

Bryan Smith

Introduction

The phrase 'outdoor education and residential experience' contains two elements which are complementary and in practice frequently linked. Outdoor education may provide the stimulating environment around which hangs the rest of a residential experience. A limited period away from home creates educational opportunities which are fundamentally different from those available within one day. Taken together the combination has great potential for the personal and social development of young people.

Within the field of outdoor education and residential experience current thinking related to broader areas of education has led some teachers to recognise three significant developments:

1. A reappraisal of the learning process and the role of the student in this process.
2. The developing role of outdoor education and residential experience as an integral element of the curriculum.
3. The increasing need for effective management of a complex aspect of educational provision.

The latter two developments are, I feel, a consequence of the potential offered by the first. I would therefore like to concentrate attention on the learning process and the corresponding role of the student. A theoretical approach is balanced against related developments within the practice of outdoor education and residential experience. As it is an area of education which falls across the curriculum rather than existing within defined curriculum areas there are implications for many subject areas.

The learning process and the role of the student

By involvement in concrete experiences in which a sense of personal success is felt, self-esteem and self-confidence are likely to increase. Residential and outdoor experiences, for young people in particular, can be sufficiently influential to act as significant reference points for future behaviour, standing out from other less easily recollected events. Reflection on these experiences in a social setting in which there is an environment of trust can lead to greater self-disclosure and a greater willingness to take responsibility for personal behaviour. By taking greater responsibility for one's own behaviour there is an improved relationship between oneself, others and the environment of which we are all part. These are qualities which are integral to the personal and social development of young people and outdoor and residential education is one means by which they may be nourished.

Much of the growth in the use of the outdoor environment for educational purposes during the last 25 years will be justified in similar terms to the above. The primary reasons for introducing large numbers of young people to adventurous activities, rock climbing, canoeing, orienteering, gorge walking or camping for example have been to help promote the personal and social development of those young people (Schools' Council, 1980). Even those teachers concerned with residential field courses linked to syllabus requirements for examination have adopted such aims in an increasingly overt manner (Geographical Association, 1984). The outdoor pursuit course, fieldwork or foreign language exchange visit will feature as a clear recollection in the minds of the participants for many years to come.

There is now, however, a great range of educationally-based outdoor and residential experiences offered to young people through, for example, the Youth Training Scheme, City Technical Colleges or Technical and Vocational Education. Some independent organisations, such as Outward Bound, offer educationally-based outdoor and residential experiences on an urban or rural basis. Groups involved in urban adventure may make use of more accessible and familiar environments including greater use of school grounds. Indoor aspects of residential experience may form an integral part of a course, in planning or reviewing outdoor activities, or may indeed be justified in themselves as with the use of drama, photography, artwork, discussion, social work or games and simulations. Adventurous experiences are more frequently linked to environmental awareness and the ethics of conservation. The age, ability levels and cultural backgrounds from which participants are drawn is widening and includes many with special needs. Environmental education now incorporates many more subject headings which make use of the outdoor environment, shown by the Schools' Council 'Art in the built environment' or the 13–16 history syllabus.

What recent common developments can be recognised in all of the above? It is a questioning of how people learn. Outdoor and residential education offers a potential for young people to learn in forms not easily available.

The ideas developed here relate primarily to experiential learning (Lewin, 1951) and consequently to aspects of social learning theory (Bandura, 1977). The emphasis is on process in education rather than content, and developing the ability to reflect on meaningful personal experience and on the modelled behaviour others provide in social circumstances. Aspects of the outdoor and residential experience can approximate to the peak experience identified by Maslow (1971).

Experiential learning

In the Lewinian experiential learning model a cyclical representation of the learning process is described and encompasses a process that Lewin (1951) considers most effectively facilitates personal growth. The model represented in Figure 6.1 is from Kolb (1984), who refers to Lewin, Dewey and Piaget as providing the intellectual origins of experiential learning.

As Newman (1986) emphasises it does not matter where the starting point is in the cycle, provided all four stages are experienced.

A number of characteristics of experiential learning can be identified which are instrumental in determining the effectiveness of outdoor and residential education. By recognising these characteristics a clearer guide to future practice may be established.

DESIGN OF THE EXPERIENCE
There is participant involvement in the design of the experience. The individual therefore has a greater degree of responsibility for their own learning. The individual participates in the

116

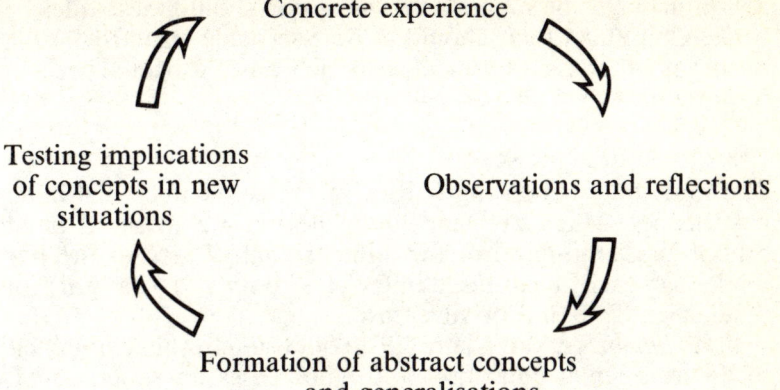

Figure 6.1 *Cyclical model of experiential learning*

decision-making process which governs the nature of the subsequent experience.

Outdoor education frequently involves young people taking part in experiences exclusively planned by adults and teaching staff. This need not be the case. There can be opportunities for whole group discussion and decision making at all stages, provided the experience is pitched at the level of those taking part. It requires a flexible attitude of those involved about the eventual outcome of the experience, if others are to have their say.

If the teacher is deciding on a camp site to stay at, the students can easily be involved in the decision. Alternatives may be presented to the group, bearing in mind distance, weather conditions, the site and individual levels of ability. Members of the group should have an opportunity to make their feelings known.

Equally, they can be involved in budgeting and liaison or gathering appropriate items of equipment. The Field Studies Council have recently run courses for TVEI groups which involve students keeping to a budget for their teaching resources and 'buying in' staff as needed to carry out a range of tasks.

Contracts or less formal agreements can be drawn up prior to a group living together at a youth hostel, for instance. Rules with regard to smoking or visiting the local town are more likely to be adhered to if previously discussed and agreed to. Appropriate action may also be suggested by the group should these rules be broken. Similarly there should be time set aside regularly for the airing of other issues and ideas which any individual feels is important.

CONCRETE EXPERIENCES

The individual is personally involved in concrete or first-hand experiences. Much of what young people are involved in at school is second-hand or two dimensional. Which of the five senses can easily be aroused in the classroom and what sense of scale, friendship, fun or adventure?

In *Acclimatizing*, Van-Matre (1974) offers a refreshing approach to environmental education and emphasises an experimental approach to all of the above-mentioned senses. Through sensory exploration the focus is on involvement, discovery, imagination and enthusiasm. It is an approach which aims to build a relationship based on understanding and feeling between the individual and the natural world.

The issue of conservation interests many young people and features in a large number of syllabuses. It is possible to learn of the need for conservation from slides, text-books and the television. If, however, young people are actively involved in conservation tasks the issues are more clearly understood and there is a greater likelihood of future independent involvement. Community projects involving tree planting schemes, pond clearance or the design of murals may get across the message that conservation begins at home.

However, learning by doing is only part of the process. A walk in the hills with a group of young people will not, automatically, be a valuable learning experience. It depends on the particular aims and objectives of the activity which need to be established beforehand, yet allow for spontaneity.

REFLECTION

There is an opportunity to reflect on the experience. This element is, I feel, most important and involves a skill which needs to be developed in young people. Reflection may involve many different complementary processes. Independent thought about contemporary experiences does not necessarily come easily to adolescents or adults.

Spragg (1984) lists activities which illustrate that 'reflection is not just a discussion'. Reflection is an activity which may take place immediately following an activity or many years later. It not only enables people to draw out of an experience what they have learnt but critically promotes a questioning process whereby personal decisions are more effectively made.

The use of a video camera or photographs allows a whole group to focus their attention on one particular event in which they took part. How much more illuminating it is to look at how your group solved the 'acid stream problem' if viewed on the television and consequently to discuss how people worked together.

A group diary formed during a residential period encourages collective reflection and may include sketches, cartoons, photographs or commentary. A word processor allows a professional finish which, with subsequent duplication, provides a permanent and attractive record.

Personal reviewing and recording, profiling and records of achievement are all variants on the significant development of documenting aspects of outdoor education and residential experience for the benefit of the individual and other interested parties. If an individual demonstrates skills or abilities previously unrecorded it seems to me that we have a duty to recognise these positive achievements in a permanent record of some sort.

Davies and Gibson (1967, p 106) question whether a transfer of learning takes place for young people from adventurous outdoor activities to 'their everyday life'. I would say that transfers of learning are enhanced if there is an opportunity for reflection. Otherwise the experience may be enjoyable and exciting but ephemeral.

TRUST AND EMPATHY

If the reflection involves others an atmosphere of trust and empathy is important. The work of Rogers (1983) is important in emphasising the need for empathy, positive regard and genuineness in a constructive learning environment.

If a group forms for only five or ten days away from home there is limited time for the development of relationships from which individual growth may spring. None the less even in this limited period close relationships of trust and understanding can certainly grow and no doubt account for the value of residential education.

More can be made of the residential experience however if

those group areas formed in schools, tutor groups, subjected groups and friendship groups are able to build on the elements of trust and empathy which already exist within the group, prior to, during and after the residential aspect of the experience. This involves members of staff as well as students and stresses the importance of cohesive groups staying together throughout a residential experience.

CONTROL
The individual has a measure of control over the experience. While conditions may dictate that other principles take precedence, that the possible price of failure is too high for example, the element of control should be allowed to move towards the child as previous learning experiences are consolidated and developed. Whatever methods are used within residential activities, there should be planned progression from greater control by staff to independence of action by the young people concerned.

A fieldwork experiment will be much more meaningful to the student if he or she is allowed to take responsibility for its design and implementation with later evaluation. Mistakes of course will be made but the learning which results will be all the greater if appropriate guidance is given. Indeed GCSE and 'A' level syllabuses frequently illustrate this attitude of individual responsibility. The greater danger is that teachers do too much of the work for the students.

BUILDING ON EXPERIENCE
There is an opportunity to build on the initial experience. Additional experiences are built on the concepts and generalisations formed from previous experience. The cycle of experiential learning is in fact a spiral.

Do we provide opportunities for all to build on their early experiences or are there barriers which restrict the participation of some individuals? I am thinking here of non-swimmers being ineligible to take part in water-based courses, of residential courses offered to pupils whose parents prevent them from attending for cultural reasons, those disqualified by financial circumstances or activities which imply a high level of physical ability. Are alternatives offered? In recent years I believe there has been a much greater awareness of the value of providing out-

120

door and residential experiences for all so that each person may build on their own previous experience in a structured way.

MOTIVATION

There is greater motivation to repeat positive experiences. Failure is a disincentive to learn. Glasser (1969) considered that the major problems of schools is one of failure in which many experiences are negative and down putting. Psychologically we seek experiences which are enjoyable and stimulating and which we do not view negatively. However, this does not invalidate learning experiences which incorporate failure or short-fall. With reflection the lessons learnt from any sense of failure may be put to positive use.

Residential education easily allows activities to be incorporated that show young people how they may succeed in their own eyes and those of others. As a result confidence grows and they wish to repeat these activities or attempt to explore other areas: steering a narrow boat, for example; ordering a ticket in French; living away from home or completing a rock climb.

The points raised here are equally applicable to the ordinary school environment if the overall methods of approach are altered. Out of that environment, however, there is greater freedom from constraints. The atmosphere is generally more informal than that of schools, time is less precisely organised, opportunities are readily available for relationships to form, a flexibility in approach is readily accepted and the environment is frequently a stimulating one. It is for these reasons, I believe, that many teachers and young people take opportunities which are available outside the classroom. There are also greater professional and individual risks involved, because of the absence of some of the above constraints.

Outdoor and residential education is fundamentally a social experience over an extended period where the behaviour of others in a range of stimulating environments provides a model whereby an individual may evaluate the efficacy of future behaviour. The role of peer group influences and modelling for adolescents explains the great potential for the secondary age group.

Young people in a social setting primarily learn by observing others and either immediately or subsequently adapting that information for use by themselves. Learning by doing, which is an oversimplification for experiential learning, is generally not a

121

trial and error process but is the method by which the individual personally adapts to the messages and impressions he has picked up from other people.

In residential situations this is seen to be the case all the time. Watch a group of young people or adults trying on items of equipment for the first time, taking part in a discussion, doing the washing up or sitting in a canoe and they are invariably watching each other at the same time. Each of the above are relatively straightforward tasks. They are not only picking up a skill, by observation followed by immediate personal experience, but learning patterns of behaviour in a social sense; how people react to each other and themselves. Importantly, Bandura (1977) emphasises, that people also notice the consequences of this behaviour, and how it is viewed by others. Is the behaviour socially rewarded or punished? Clearly previously experienced patterns of behaviour will have a bearing on how people react. They adapt, with new experience, to the different circumstances as well as to different personalities.

Furthermore, people learn most from those events which capture their attention and which they are then able to retain as striking images. Also, by definition, they learn from the people they are most frequently with but from some individuals more than others. The learning potential of a group of strangers is likely to be less than that of a group of friends. There is an element of experimenting, adapting and transferring the observed behaviour of others. The process of modelling social skills, such as making a newcomer to the group feel welcome, may be equally complex.

A group building a raft together produces a multitude of exchanges, of messages and communications. People step forward or hesitate, more or less watching others and listening to their comments. There is a 'to-ing and fro-ing' of active involvement and reflection. With later reflection the learning process may be drawn out more clearly. By helping to create experiences in which the outcomes are positive, which result in success not failure, where people feel valued for what they contribute, the resulting modelled behaviour is also more likely to be adopted.

Peer group influences and modelling, I suggest, are very significant for adolescents and are likely to be prominent in the intense environment of a residential setting. It seems that during adolescence there is an unusual sensitivity to the statements members of the peer group make about any member of that group (Elder, 1968). This is particularly the case with friends.

The peak experiences of 'awe, mystery, wonder or of perfect completion' of which Maslow (1971, p 197) writes are not uncommon within groups of young people away from home. Reflecting on those experiences can be an empowering force leading to greater individual autonomy. The kinds of triggers available to produce a peak experience are frequent in unfamiliar environments. It may be a bivouac at midnight, a narrow boat at dawn, climbing in a dramatic mountain environment or talking to a friend with an intensity not previously felt. The 24-hour journey, planned to encompass a variety of activities, may incorporate a number of peak experiences, in a group setting or individually. These can be powerful and complex emotional and personal movements, powerful learning experiences.

It is the peak experiences, or those that approximate to that state, to which I feel we most easily return, in our mind's eye. It can be a time of attitude changes, of seeing things from a new perspective, a freshening of experience (Maslow, 1964, p 78).

Conclusion

Those teachers involved in outdoor education and residential experience contribute significantly to the provision of a great range of learning experiences for young people. Reflecting on the principles which guide practice and on the associated styles of work which are adopted can only enrich the curriculum which is offered.

I have tried, therefore, to put the practice of outdoor and residential education on a firmer theoretical footing. Our understanding of how people learn has developed enormously in recent years and unless we are to stand still new ways of working need to be considered. Outdoor and residential experiences can offer considerable learning opportunities for young people. I have tried to show how people involved may be able to make more of those opportunities.

References

Bandura, A (1977) *Social Learning Theory* Prentice Hall, New Jersey.
Davies, B and Gibson, A (1967) *The Social Education of the Adolescent* University of London, London.

Elder, G (1968) Adolescent socialisation and development, in E Borgatta and W Lambert (eds.), *Handbook of Personality Theory and Research* Rand McNally.

Geographical Association Sixth Form/University Working Party (1984) The enduring purpose of fieldwork, *Teaching Geography*, 9, (5).

Glasser, W (1969) *Schools without Failure* Harper and Row, London.

Kolb, D (1984) *Experiential Learning* Prentice Hall, London.

Lewin, K (1951) *Field Theory in Social Sciences* Harper and Row, London.

Maslow, A (1964) *Religions, Values and Peak Experiences* Ohio State University Press, Columbus.

Maslow, A (1971) *The Farther Reaches of Human Nature*, Pelican, London.

Newman, G (1986) 14+ choices – causes for concern, *Educational Management and Administration*, 14, 145–52.

Rogers, C R (1983) *Freedom to Learn in the 80s* Harper and Row, London.

Schools' Council (1980) *Outdoor Education in Secondary Schools* Schools' Council, London.

Spragg, D (1984) Learning to learn, *Adventure Education* 1 (1).

Van-Matre, S (1974) *Acclimatizing* American Camping Association, Indiana.

Part 3

Introduction

In Part 3 aspects of the whole school curriculum are related to physical education. Chapter 7 examines the contribution of physical education to the health promoting school. In the proposals for a national curriculum, health education is seen as a 'theme' in which different subject areas make their unique contributions and the staff within the school are responsible for ensuring that a coherent message is provided for young people. There are some dangers in this approach, especially with the move towards modularisation of the curriculum, because coherence and specific features of health education, for example role of energy balance in controlling weight, can easily be lost unless some form of careful monitoring is instigated to ensure that all pupils have access to a core of health experiences.

In the same way, the unique contributions of subjects like physical education, with their concern for health related exercise, have to make strong representation in meetings about curriculum policy decisions. If this does not happen an important aspect of health education may be lost. Thus, all of the staff in physical education departments have to be aware of their unique contributions to health education and understand the implications when planning their programmes for the coming year.

Chapter 7 makes the point that physical education staff have a unique contribution to make in the area of health and suggests how this can be brought about. There is no suggestion that this aspect of physical education should take over from all the other important features of a sound balanced programme and dominate a teacher's time and energies. However, the proposals in this chapter require careful reading because a health concern does entail a change of focus and the inherent messages need to be understood if one is to be faithful to its principles.

There is a lot to learn and much to appreciate in the principles underlying a change of focus to take on board health concerns in physical education. Jo Harris provides much food for thought in her explanations of what could be involved in a focus on health. Underpinning a commitment to health and life-style is the need for young people to learn to be responsible for their life-style decisions and accept such a responsibility. Here, the implications for physical education really bite because young people need the opportunity in their curriculum time to learn this message and experience situations which help them acquire this disposition. This will not be easy for many physical education staff but the will is there for them to learn. On the other hand, the need to teach a concern for being responsible is a whole school concern reinforced in the way that individual subject areas plan curriculum experiences.

The change of focus in physical education which is being proposed in all the chapters in this book is closely associated with a concern for personal and social development in the curriculum. The content changes being proposed in games, athletics, swimming, gymnastics, and outdoor adventure education are directly related to a need to personalise educational experiences, not in some egalitarian sense but in terms of relevance and significance to every pupil.

The concern for responsibility in making decisions about health related exercise in one's life-style is important in one's learning, but also in one's conduct. In the idea of sport education morally acceptable attitudes and conduct are seen as an important aspect of a physical education programme. Here, the disgraceful scenes of violence and unacceptable social behaviour of certain sporting fans as they follow their teams in European countries illustrate the need to teach young people about morally acceptable attitudes. Freedom and responsibility in advancing one's leisure need to be associated with recognising the rights and welfare of others and not as in soccer violence where the freedom of others is diminished and where pleasure is derived only at the expense of others. I would argue strongly that schools have an important role to play in educating young people to recognise unacceptable sporting behaviour and it is here that physical education staff need to be associated with personal and social education.

Chapter 8 attempts to sketch out a framework for considering personal and social education in physical education. Len Almond proposes that this aspect of physical education is not something that is caught in the process of taking part in different sporting activities, gymnastics, or adventure pursuits, instead it is something that has to be carefully planned to ensure that experiences, which promote personal development and social education, are a fundamental part of a young person's physical education, and recognised as such by staff. An assumption that personal and social education is caught and not planned means that teachers are ignoring the potential of their subject, but also it means that teachers see themselves only as teachers of specific activities in a kind of technical sense.

Personal and social education like health education is a kind of theme that different subject areas contribute towards. However, if schools are to develop a coherent strategy for personal and social education as a cross-curricular theme then it is important for physical education teachers to recognise their contribution and acknowledge their role in its promotion. Chapter 8 on personal and social education, attempts to do this so that physical education teachers can develop the potential of their subject and also play a significant role in the whole curriculum as well. The uniqueness of physical education's contribution to the curriculum must be acknowledged but its role in cross-curricular links has also to be recognised.

Finally, Chapter 9 'Accreditation', provides an insight into some of the developments beginning to emerge in the 14–18 curriculum. It is here that major developments in the school curriculum are starting to force a change of thinking in physical education. At present the rethinking process has hit many further education establishments but teachers in secondary schools have started to consider the implications.

The notion of accreditation is closely linked at present to certification but this can be extended and it would have far-reaching implications.

Teachers who have introduced GCSE have had to engage in planning courses for approval, collaborate in moderating standards and this experience has had an important spin-off. Physical education staff not involved in examination-based courses have not been required to put together a course structure and there has been no accountability to ensure that this has been completed. It is my opinion that this neglect has led many teachers to back away from curriculum development in physical education because it has involved a large element of planning and a commitment to writing down course content in detail.

Thus, the accreditation of courses in physical education would involve staff in planning courses for approval as part of a school-based certificate, a local cluster of schools, an LEA panel, or national initiatives. The modularisation of the 14–16 curriculum would speed up this process and contribute directly to the abolition of recreation-type options which have dominated much of physical education in the recent past. Many young people involved in recreation-type activities are not being taught and I firmly believe that there is no longer any room for this kind of programme. Bernard Dickenson's analysis of accreditation and his description of what could be included provides a major debating point which will dominate much of our thinking in physical education.

Many teachers will argue that there is a need to maintain the practical commitment of physical education and if this is lost the profession is denigrating its responsibilities. There is a mistaken belief that proposals for accreditation will involve some form of theoretical study. The suggestions for TVEI and GCSE courses involving physical education are far from theoretical studies and the sooner teachers can see examples of these courses the better. Dickenson's example of the Midland Record of Achievement illustrates something of the movement towards accreditation and though it is only one example of achievements that could contribute to pupil profiles, it provides a good example of how traditional courses can be modified and accredited.

The three chapters in this part illustrate the changing face of physical education as its contribution to the whole curriculum becomes problematic. Teachers of physical education have been seeking guidance in this area for sometime, therefore these chapters can provide the basis for much discussion and reflection.

Chapter 7
A Health Focus in Physical Education

Jo Harris

Introduction

A concern for health in physical education has surfaced once again. In this chapter I propose to outline some of the benefits of health related exercise and provide a framework for considering how teachers of physical education can highlight ways in which a health focus can become a feature of their programmes.

Why a health focus in physical education?

The health benefits of exercise have been well established (Fentem *et al*, 1988) over the years and it is clear that regular and appropriate physical activity can promote:

- an improved functional capacity;
- a more efficient cardiovascular system;
- an increase in mineral content and greater mechanical strength of bones (which aids growth and development of the skeleton and helps to offset osteoporosis);
- the development of muscle fitness (important to joint stability and sound posture);
- better control of, and more desirable, body weight; and
- enhanced mental functioning (feelings of well-being, increased self-esteem and reduced stress levels).

Indeed, regular exercise not only promotes the healthy functioning of various body systems but can also exert a protective effect against heart disease by influencing favourably such risk factors as overweight, hypertension and harmful blood fat levels. It has even been suggested that inactivity is almost comparable to a high cholesterol level, high blood pressure, or smoking a pack of cigarettes a day as a risk factor for coronary heart disease which is currently the biggest killer in the western world.

There is little doubt then that regular exercise is a positive health habit and most people would agree that exercise is good for them. Yet many adults, young people and children reveal a pattern of inactivity and lack of regular, vigorous exercise outside of school hours. It is also known that in Britain children spend on average about three hours a day watching television (Tuxworth, 1988). Further evidence is accumulating that the course of events leading to heart disease begins in childhood and adolescence. Such findings have led to the current concern about the physical inactivity of many children and young people and this concern has been expressed by representatives from exercise science, physiology, child health, community medicine, education and sport. The overwhelming message is that it is desirable and necessary for all children and young people to engage in frequent, appropriate exercise.

Schools alone cannot take responsibility for activating the nation. It is important to recognise that at a local level the promotion of exercise is a joint venture between home, school and the community. On a wider scale, it is essential that relevant national organisations continue to highlight the health benefits of exercise and ultimately, it is hoped that the government will come round to accepting the fact that the country needs an exercise campaign!

What is a focus on health?

If one accepts that the current provision for exercise in schools cannot, by itself, be sufficient to compensate for the out-of-school inactivity levels of children, what is it that schools can do to promote active life-styles? First, schools can accept that they are in a position to favourably influence the behaviour patterns of young people and should consider formulating an exercise policy for the whole school. Second, those responsible for the physical education curriculum need to consider whether the curriculum provides opportunities for enhancing the necessary affective, cognitive, motor and social skills essential for lifetime involvement in physical activity. The priority here should be to develop long-term positive attitudes towards physical activity rather than short-term transient changes in physiological status. There is little to be gained from winning one battle yet ultimately losing the war.

Young children generally like to move, play, run, climb and jump. However, somewhere between childhood and puberty, these children turn towards a life-style of inactivity. In fact, some teachers and coaches may have reinforced inactivity by using physical activity as a punishment – we can probably all think of someone who has used sit-ups or running laps to punish wrongdoers. Maybe a more appropriate strategy would be to reprimand a pupil by asking them to sit still and not to move! Fortunately, physical educators have moved a long way in their thinking and 'exercise as aversion therapy' – the old 'blood, sweat and tears' approach – has hopefully been put to rest.

It should be a priority of physical educators to build and reinforce positive attitudes towards physical activity. This necessitates developing a positive health focus in physical education emphasising the fact that health-related exercise is for all and that physical education is for life. In order that the latter notion should not seem like a life sentence, it is vital that the curriculum offers pupils enjoyable and satisfying exercise experiences. These experiences should be varied with some activities involving periods of short-duration intense exercise as with traditional games, while others should constitute more prolonged lower-intensity exercise, for example swimming, running, rope-skipping, exercise to music, walking, and dancing. There should also be a balance of skill-related competitive activities and more health-related lifetime activities.

If pupils' experience of physical education is one which they find satisfying and generates good feelings, it is likely that they will wish to repeat these experiences more frequently. Further, young people need to feel that they are capable of taking part and have the confidence to participate fully. They will only be motivated towards further participation if they experience a sense of achievement and accomplishment through physical activity. An over-emphasis on skill-related activities for a significant number of pupils, may well be counter-productive in promoting active life-styles.

An emphasis on pupil-centred and individualised learning should help children and young people to appreciate that health benefits through exercise are attainable and worthwhile goals for everyone. Everyone can feel good about their performance since recognition of progress and improvement comes from within. Fitness is not the exclusive right of elite performers – everyone can be fitter and healthier than the person they were yesterday. However, it must be emphasised that health and wellness have to be achieved – they cannot be worked on just for a few weeks in order to store the benefits, and picked up again when the mood suits one. Good health and physical well-being are achievements that only come about because people incorporate frequent physical activity into their life-style and maintain it on a regular basis.

A major feature of a concern for a health focus in physical education is the promotion of active life-styles. This involves promoting physical activity as a good experience, showing a concern for raising pupil self-esteem through exercise, and helping pupils learn how to incorporate positive health behaviours into their life-style. It is undoubtedly a challenge to motivate young people to exercise regularly. The gauntlet has been thrown down and physical educators are encouraged to accept the challenge boldly. There is still much to be learnt about factors affecting exercise adherence, but it will be a major step forward if we can get the vast majority of our pupils looking forward to their physical education lessons and enjoying some form of exercise, not simply because it is a break from academic work. It is vital that children retain their early delight in physical activity and play, and that the exercise habit is continued into adolescence and adulthood.

The provision of enjoyable and satisfying exercise experiences within the curriculum can easily be supplemented by encouraging pupils to:

- increase their routine activity levels (for example, cycling to school, climbing stairs, walking to town rather than taking the bus);
- join in some of the extra-curricular activities offered at school;
- consider joining some of the local sports clubs;
- take up some of the opportunities offered at the local sports centres; and
- exercise at home;

The implications for physical education teachers are that they:

- respect individuals;

- take note of and show interest in what pupils do;
- praise effort; and
- continue to encourage and motivate.

In addition, if pupils are to be encouraged sincerely to join in school clubs at lunchtime and after school, it is necessary that the extra-curricular programme offers opportunities for all ability levels. Is this the case?

Further, does the programme offer what the pupils want? If you are not sure, don't be afraid to ask! Young people can come up with some good ideas – all the better if they are also willing to help organise activities, scout for new members and maybe even run the activities themselves. After all, meeting pupils' needs and encouraging independence are what schools are all about.

An increase in routine activity and out-of-school exercise can be prompted with the use of activity diaries, exercise log sheets and the setting up of clubs such as the 100-mile club in which pupils attempt to participate in 100 miles of aerobic activity over a specified time such as a school term.

These ideas not only aid motivation but also create links with the home and community and help pupils to appreciate that exercise habits are an important part of one's life-style and not just something which they experience while at school.

In addition to promoting active life-styles, a second feature of a concern for a health focus in physical education is the need for young people to acquire a practical knowledge base so that they acquire knowledge and understanding of the way the body responds to exercise. There is a need for young people to learn the How, the What and the Why of exercise so that they understand what they are doing and why they are doing it, and have the necessary skills to put it into practice. There is much to be learnt about performing exercise in a correct manner, how much exercise is relevant, when it can be developed, and how it can be incorporated successfully into one's life experiences and routines. The following questions are examples of those which need addressing: What exercises are safe to do? Are there any exercises I should avoid? How do I know if I'm exercising hard enough? What kinds of activities are best for me? How often should I exercise? For how long should I exercise? Which activities will help me lose weight? What should I do before and after exercising? Do I need to be fit to play sports? I'm very unfit – where should I start? How much exercise is enough? These are important questions and pupils need the answers in order to be intelligent exercise performers and knowledgeable fitness consumers.

Physical education programmes need to incorporate planned learning alongside practical work. The practical knowledge base is too important to be left to incidental teaching and should be available to all pupils and not just those in examination groups or the more able performers who are seen more frequently at extra-curricular activities. The knowledge gained is practical in the sense that it is applied and physical in the sense that it is all about action. A practical knowledge base could be described as knowledge acquired 'through action for action' where young people can demonstrate that they 'know and understand'. The emphasis is thus on experiential learning where young people learn through 'doing'.

The development of a health focus in physical education does not imply a reduction in physical activity and an immense increase in theoretical work. Indeed many concepts, such as the effects of exercise intensity on breathing rate and heart rate, can be taught by means of practical workcards where groups of pupils are guided through appropriate practical activities and the theoretical knowledge gained through the experience of doing the activity. The Health and Physical Education Project team based at Loughborough University and funded by the Health Education Authority are soon to publish resource materials for teachers which will include a 12-lesson introductory teaching programme entitled 'Action for heart health'. Future materials will deal with other health-related areas such as posture and back-care, flexibility, muscle fitness and the stress factor. These publications will provide numerous tried and tested teaching ideas for blending theory and practice in an enjoyable and informative manner.

Integrating a health focus into physical education

How should this knowledge base be incorporated into the curriculum? First, the traditional physical education programme of games, athletics, dance, gymnastics and swimming provides much scope for teaching pupils about how to exercise safely and correctly and how to acquire health benefits through exercise. In some curriculum areas there is a specific emphasis, which is central to the activity and which can contribute to an overall focus on health. Thus, in gymnastics, strength and flexibility are key components, whereas in swimming and athletics endurance or aerobic exercise have a significant place, and in dance there is an opportunity for all of these areas to be developed, plus work on posture and relaxation. There are, therefore, opportunities within the traditional programme to highlight specific features of exercise. The task for the teacher is to identify which aspects of the knowledge base are appropriate for particular pupil groups and where this can be most effectively transmitted within the curriculum. In order that a health focus is not lost, it is important that the teacher set aside time within a particular curriculum activity where the emphasis can be highlighted and pupils recognise its significance. In this way the practical knowledge base is not seen as a mere spin-off, but as a deliberate emphasis.

However, over the years, there is a great deal for a pupil to learn which cannot be taught easily within the traditional activity-based curriculum, therefore it is necessary to introduce a new type of course. A health-focus perspective calls for specific modules which can be taught alongside sport-based courses. These modules must stand in their own right and be practically based rather than theoretical courses. Within these modules, pupils can gain valuable knowledge about cardiovascular health, flexibility, muscle fitness, posture and back-care, stress and relaxation, exercise programmes and life-style management. They can also experience a variety of safe and correct exercises and aerobic activities such as walking, jogging, running, rope skipping, exercise to music, dancing, swimming, and, where possible, cycling. These so-called 'lifetime' activities tend to be very much undervalued within conventional physical education programmes. There are also numerous ways in which traditional games can be modified and new games created to emphasise continuous activity for all participants within a structured yet enjoyable setting.

'Health' has very wide parameters and in some schools still tends to be 'everyone's concern but nobody's responsibility'. There is no suggestion that the physical education curriculum should take on board all facets of health education. Indeed many health issues would probably be best incorporated in other curriculum areas and the ideal situation would be for a school to have an established health policy and/or exercise policy involving a high degree of co-operation and integration between different departments or faculties.

Much valuable work can be covered in traditional health education lessons or within the personal and social education programme. For example, young people can learn to: recognise the value of exercise in their life-style; become aware of some of the barriers to exercise participation (social, time, economics, environment, knowledge of facilities, access) and develop strategies to help tackle these and incorporate exercise into their life experiences and routines. In the upper school, TVEI, B Tech (Foundation Studies) courses, GCSE and modular studies provide further opportunities for valuable cross-curricular links. Modules entitled 'Life-style management', 'Healthy living' and 'Health skills' are just some examples of courses which could be offered and which can reinforce the message that exercise is a valuable contributor to health.

A further development of a health focus in physical education might be to move beyond a health re-emphasis within the traditional activity-based courses or new modules, towards the idea that, as a health promoting school, special events or promotions could be planned to involve the community. A physical activity week, a healthy heart day, a 'low-stress, high-relaxation' (or 'cool-it!') day or a healthy eating day could provide opportunities for highlighting the value of an active life-style and for school and community organisations to work together on a joint enterprise. Such events emphasise the importance of support structures in terms of the home, school and the community, effectively promoting and reinforcing the health message.

Developing a health focus within physical education will necessarily involve adopting a variety of teaching styles. A pupil-centred and personalised approach is most appropriate with teachers encouraging pupils to become more responsible for their own learning. The health message is about making informed choices and being responsible for one's own actions. Thus, it is important that this opportunity is made available to young people in the physical education programme so that they can learn to be responsible and make their own decisions. Unfortunately, most people regard health in a negative context as a possession which alleviates illness and implies absence from disease. It is important, therefore, that health is put across in a positive context to help young people appreciate that they have some control over what they choose to do and that good health and wellness have to be achieved. It is also important that young people value the role of regular exercise in enhancing physical well-being and appreciate its potential for enhancing the quality of life. It is suggested that a more appropriate and workable definition of health might be:

Health is not a static condition, existing only in the absence of disease, but is an ongoing process of learning, decision making, and action for optimising one's well-being.

In summary, it is believed that the physical education curriculum should reflect the following two essential concerns:

1 Physical education is for all.
2 Physical education is for life.

Further, a positive health focus within the physical education curriculum has to be deliberately planned in order to:

- promote active life-styles; and
- provide a practical knowledge base.

The focus for an active life-style should be on:

- promoting physical activity as an enjoyable and satisfying experience;
- a concern for raising pupil self-esteem through exercise; and
- developing pupils' awareness of the choices they can make in terms of exercise behaviour and life-style habits.

The focus for a practical knowledge base should be on:

- providing opportunities for gaining knowledge and understanding in terms of exercise and its effects on the body;
- experiential learning situations in which pupils learn through 'doing'; and
- encouraging pupils to take greater responsibility for their own exercise behaviour thus leading them from dependence to independence.

Finally, it is worth emphasising that the development of a health focus in physical education is highly desirable and should be encouraged, not simply because of the alarmingly high coronary heart disease figures in this country, but more importantly to:

- contribute towards good health, physical well-being and a feeling of wellness;
- enhance the quality of life; and
- provide energy to enrich life.

The challenge is an exciting one – let us take it on board and ensure that, for our pupils, PE represents a Positive Experience rather than Pain and Earache!

References

Fentem, P, Bassey, J and Turnbull, N B (1988) *The New Case for Exercise* Health Education Authority, London.

Tuxworth, W (1988) The fitness and physical activity of adolescents, *The Medical Journal of Australia*, **148**, 513–21.

Chapter 8

Developing Personal and Social Skills within Physical Education

Len Almond

Introduction

In this chapter I shall assume a position in which, if I was a Head of a school with the full support of the physical education staff, I would like to propose a framework for fostering personal and social education. Thus, I am adopting to some extent an idealist position by proposing a framework for a school that I would like to see. However, my proposals provide the means to consider their significance and to explore the potential role of personal and social education in physical education, and to assess how far such aspirations can be translated into learning opportunities. In both cases, this framework provides the means for going beyond a general review of literature on the topic, and seeing a practical exemplar of what personal and social education could look like in physical education. I have deliberately left out of the title the word development, because this takes me into a realm which is best handled by psychologists who are prepared to provide guidelines for teachers, or enter into a liaison to plan personal and social education programmes to ensure continuity and development.

In order to create a framework to characterise personal and social education I propose to use two components which form the basis for developing a more elaborate structure.

Content

The content that we present to young people should be a personal encounter in which young people learn to recognise the need for mastery to enhance the satisfactions derived from engagement in purposeful physical activity. However, teachers

139

need to acknowledge also that this will only come about if pupils have something to gain (it is personally rewarding) from taking part in physical activity, and where success can be seen as attainable. So often success in physical education can be attributed to maturational factors, and when one considers that social comparison is used as the process by which individuals gauge their success (or failure), it is little wonder that many pupils do not find it intrinsically rewarding. This requires the teacher to redefine what counts as success in physical education and identify indicators which reward effort and achievement over time and as far as possible are independent of maturational factors. Thus, there is a need for a shift in focus to ensure that the degree of achievement over time rather than ability to perform – or maturational factors – is the basis for indicating success.

The self-esteem of an individual will play an important role in supporting mastery and reinforcing the satisfactions to be gained from achievement.

Associated with this concern for mastery and the personalising of experience is the need to promote the idea that everyone can be good at exercising, so that pupils do not use their performance and achievements in sport, which may be poor, as the basis for estimating their capability to exercise. Also, underpinning a concern for mastery is the need to recognise dispositions that support learning, like concentration, perseverance, consistency, and confidence. These need to be promoted and attention paid to their acquisition for all pupils.

The opportunity for young people to discuss and critically reflect about the role of purposeful physical activity in enhancing the quality of life is an important aspect of personal development. It enables young people to acquire some understanding of what to do with their lives and provides an opportunity for an informed choice to be made. This is an important aspect of a teacher's work because it enables young people to recognise how much control they have in their lives and appreciate the limitations of personal responsibility within society and a person's community.

Context

The context in which physical education is undertaken provides numerous opportunities for planning situations in physical education which reinforce a school concern for personal and social

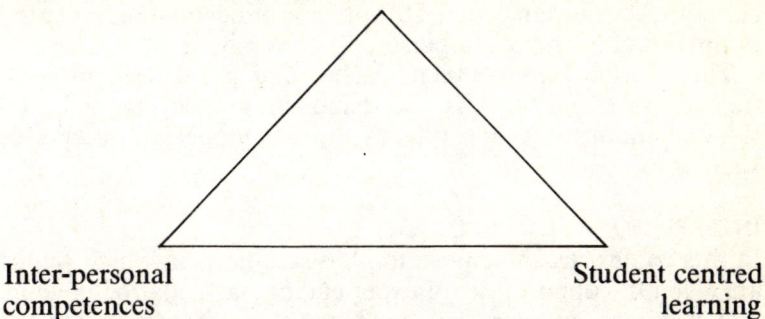

Figure 8.1 *The context in which physical education is undertaken*

education. Therefore, I would like to elaborate on three distinct aspects of the context as illustrated in Figure 8.1.

CLIMATE/ETHOS/ENVIRONMENT

This involves the way teacher expectations (Martinek *et al*, 1982) of pupil performances and acceptable behaviour, expressed in both the language they use and their visible actions during contact with pupils, influence young people in either a negative or positive manner. Young people's attitudes and behaviours are influenced by this 'hidden' curriculum, therefore teachers need to be aware of what messages they portray in their contact with pupils.

In the same way, when teachers tolerate and turn a 'blind eye' to pupil-to-pupil communications, and pupil behaviour towards other pupils, which are unacceptable or militate against mutually accepted standards, they reinforce messages from the hidden curriculum.

The rules that govern acceptable behaviour and conduct within the confines of the physical education department need to be based on a process of teacher–pupil involvement in constructing mutually acceptable codes of conduct which provide guidelines for action. These need to be acceptable within a whole school policy of conduct in which pupils have been involved in framing the guidelines. If no such school document exists, there is no reason why a physical education department should not construct its own internal guidelines document. It is important that in this process of involvement examples of 'good reasons' for each code of conduct are provided so that pupils understand why mutually acceptable codes are necessary, and they are not simply authoritarian codes. This process of negotiation is central to providing a support to personal development.

The relationships between teacher and pupil need to show trust, respect, and fairness and demonstrate a caring, and considerate atmosphere, and thereby provide models of acceptable standards.

INTERPERSONAL COMPETENCE

In this context teachers need to plan situations in which pupils are given the opportunity of experiencing particular behaviours that promote interpersonal competence and working out the implications. Within this component I recognise three aspects.

First the *social* aspect in which pair and group work enables teachers to promote:

- learning to mix with others;
- establishing relationships;
- co-operating on a task; and
- sensitivity to others.

In physical education, games making, preparing for a competition, constructing a dance and planning an adventure outing provide appropriate opportunities to develop this work. However, any form of group work or working in pairs in which pupils help each other by providing feedback on their performances give the teacher an opportunity to promote social learning in physical education. In the same way group work can be used as a process for resolving problems or moral dilemmas, and providing feedback about lessons.

Second, the *conduct* of pupils in physical education should involve:

- caring, consideration for others and unselfishness;
- trust and respect for others; and
- fairness and tolerance.

It is here that sports education can be an important medium for pursuing such dispositions. In the same way, group/pair work provides the means to develop morally acceptable attitudes and behaviour, but not as something that is simply caught in the process of teaching – it needs to be taught. At this point it is necessary to refer to Dworkin (1977), a philosopher who has written on 'rights', who makes the point that people have the right to treatment as an equal which means the right to be treated with the same respect or concern as anyone else. This is an important point for sport education.

Where it is possible, good behaviour should be reinforced and inappropriate behaviour, which is not morally or socially acceptable, should be penalised and reasons given why it is unacceptable. Once again groups or pair work can be useful in reflecting on moral dilemmas.

The major difficulty for the teacher is recognising that this is a significant aspect of education even though it means that lessons are not physically active all the time. This is a particularly significant point because there is a great deal of emphasis, and rightly so, by teacher educators in promoting an increase in pupils' active engagement on tasks and teacher effectiveness (Siedentop *et al*, 1986). The fitness movement has been interpreted by some teachers as a need for pupils to be vigorously active as much as possible. Thus, these messages are bound to create a conflict when a teacher considers the value of allowing pupils to discuss and reflect. This is a difficult lesson to be learnt for the physical education teacher.

The final aspect is that physical education provides numerous opportunities in which pupils have to learn to cope with:

- frustration in one's attempts to practise;
- the process of competition;
- success and failure in competition;
- the pressure of preparing well or meeting expectations;
- fear in gymnastics or adventure activities; and
- tension in competition or presenting a performance.

Throughout the whole of physical education young people will constantly have to face the reality of emotional upset. In practising a skill or rehearsing a dance frustration and tension can arise as one strives to get it right, or do it well. In competitions one has to learn that one cannot win all the time if one is playing worthy opponents and that the satisfactions to be derived from participation are bound up with the need to be active and the pleasure it brings. One learns to accept defeat and recognise that it is not of lasting significance and bounce back again to do one's best. In success it is important to acknowledge one's opponent as a worthy competitor who deserves one's respect (Dworkin, 1977), and not as a loser who is inferior.

In the same way that one becomes accustomed to the pressure of getting ready for the competitive moment, or getting ready to perform before an audience, one learns to tolerate the pressure that the expectations of others places on us. In gymnastics, swimming, or adventure activities young people will come face to face with situations where they experience fear and an inability to perform, tackle a challenge, or get involved. All of these situations provoke emotional reactions which young people can be taught to cope with and overcome. In learning to overcome and cope with situations it is important to have the support of a caring and safe environment in which one can react to emotional challenges and make mistakes knowing that help is available. This needs to be followed by learning to cope on one's own. These are part of the learning process and part of getting to know oneself as a person. The teacher has an important responsibility here.

STUDENT CENTRED LEARNING

In this context it needs to be recognised that the opportunity to be involved in the learning process and to acquire the competence and confidence for self-direction is important for personal education. Thus, within this aspect I recognise four components.

First, learning from doing. In this context it is important to involve the student as an active participant in the learning process rather than a passive learner who absorbs everything that a teacher presents. In this process of being active there needs to be an emphasis on planning prior to being active, but also on the reflections of one's actions in order to internalise the learning. In addition, pupils need to have the opportunity of expressing their feelings about what they have just done in order to encourage them to indicate any difficulty they are experiencing.

The second component is sharing in learning. In the first instance sharing in the learning process requires the active involvement of the pupil in what is to be learnt, but also the curriculum content, hence the need for a negotiated curriculum. In addition, this negotiation needs to be extended to deliberations about rules and codes of acceptable behaviour, and the standards that govern the life of the community within physical education should involve students so that they are mutually agreed and accepted.

However, sharing in learning involves also learning with other pupils and learning from one's peers (not just the teachers). There is much to be learnt from each other and teachers can benefit also by using feedback sheets to obtain perceptions of what pupils experience in physical education lessons, and to encourage pupils to express their ideas. In this way, pupils and teachers can learn to respect, to be sensitive and tolerant towards the variety of different perspectives that people bring to any learning situation, and to recognise that different points of view exist which need to be taken into account. It is important also that we encourage pupils to comment on each other's work and give each other teaching points to help them improve.

The third point is that within student centred learning and personal education ownership of ideas and the making of something that an individual (or group) has constructed represents a major thread. Students or pupils need to learn how to set themselves personal goals or reasonable targets, make a commitment, and strive to achieve them. It means also that pupils need to be given opportunities to make personal responses to tasks they are set in order to demonstrate the diversity of potential responses but also to indicate that each interpretation has its own individual stamp. In addition pupils need the opportunity to use their imagination to create something of their own.

Finally there is independence. In the learning process we should attempt to help pupils move from a position of dependence upon the teacher (and other pupils) for both the course of learning and what is learnt, towards independence. Thus responsibility for learning is transferred to the pupils when they learn how to assume responsibility and to be responsible for both their actions and the products of their learning. It involves also a recognition that improvement can come as one learns to take control over one's attempts to achieve.

In the context of the inter-relationships between the climate established by the teacher, the interpersonal competences that they promote, and the impact of using student centred strategies, it is possible to support and reinforce the personal emphasis of the pupils' experience of physical education and the recognition that they can achieve mastery and make progress as their increased self-esteem raises their confidence. However, this will not come about in the form of a spin-off from what teachers put into a curriculum, neither are such learnings neutral because pupils can acquire both positive or negative dispositions from such encounters; it is necessary, therefore, to plan and carefully examine ways in which the personal education of young people can be promoted.

References

Dworkin, R (1977) *Taking Rights Seriously* Harvard University Press, Cambridge, Mass.

Martinek, T J, Crowe, P B, and Rejeski, W J (1982) *Pygmalion in the Gym: Causes and Effects of Expectations in Teaching and Coaching*, Leisure Press, New York.

Siedentop, D, Mand, C and Taggart, A (1986) *Physical Education: Teaching and Curriculum Strategies for Grades 5–12*, Mayfield Publishing Company, Palo Alto.

Chapter 9
Accreditation: A Different Dimension for Physical Education

Bernard Dickenson

Introduction

At no other time has education, in all its forms, been subject to so much attention. In order to raise standards and provide a more relevant curriculum, a vast range of initiatives have been introduced and developed which are primarily concerned with affecting curriculum content and delivery. It is two features associated with these changes that form the focus of this chapter.

The first is concerned with the concept of accreditation as associated with courses of study for upper secondary school pupils and the second is the organisation and structure of curriculum content to accommodate nationally promoted initiatives, while also considering a practical model for delivery of a physical education programme.

I hope to demonstrate how the implications associated with the first of these features will lead into a review of the second as a departmental and whole school issue.

Accredited courses

The concept of accreditation is concerned with a validation process for a course of study which enables pupils or students to be given credit for their achievements by an organising body, which could be, for example, a school, an examination board or a university. The most common form of accreditation associated with schools has been through public examination courses.

Physical education has contributed to this system since the early 1970s, while the first GCE dance was introduced in 1966. However, during the last few years a whole range of PE related courses have evolved. Figure 9.1 illustrates some of these courses which have either gained or are in the process of receiving accredited status. Many of these courses have been developed to address 'gaps' in continuity of provision or perceived vocational 'training' needs. For example: CPVE courses provide students with an introduction to the 'world' of the leisure industry; B TEC courses provide an introductory or advanced route into vocational preparation for the leisure industry including a business studies core; 'A' level dance, physical education and sport studies provide a link between GCSE and degree level study; leaders awards introduce students to sports promotion, development and coaching.

1	CPVE	Health studies Sports studies Leisure studies
2	City and Guilds	Leisure and recreation (pts. 1 to 4) Health studies (centred based)
3	(a) B TEC first in leisure studies (b) B TEC diploma or certificate in leisure studies.	
4	GCSE	
	Mode 1	Physical education, dance, sport studies (mature)
	Mode 3	Leisure studies, health studies
5	'A' Level	Dance, physical education, sport studies
6	Governing body award schemes	

Figure 9.1 *Some of the physical education-related courses which are, to date, either in the process of development, at a pilot stage or have received accreditation*

Listed below are just some of the governing body award schemes which have a minimum age requirement of 16 years.

- CCPR Sports Leaders
- Badminton Leaders' Certificate

- Basketball Leaders' Award
- Mini Basketball Leaders' Award
- Netball Preliminary Teaching Award
- ASA Club Instructors' Certificate
- ASA Preliminary Teaching Award
- EVA Community Sports Leaders' Award
- FA Leaders Course

While there may be a range of different purposes for these courses, they all demonstrate the width and depth of learning that can be associated with physical education.

However, while it is pleasing to see the commitment to these developments, they also raise issues for consideration by the profession:

1. Should the 14 to 16 phase of schooling provide an introduction to the vocational features of sport, leisure and recreation? Could physical education departments contribute to careers as a cross-curricula development by introducing courses in these areas and if so do PE specialists have the expertise to deliver such courses? Would there be INSET implications?
2. Should all pupils have evidence of their achievements and experiences in physical education? If yes, then could or should this be demonstrated as GCSE PE?
3. Is it compatible to have courses in physical education at advanced and GCSE level, while also having similar level courses in what are normally considered to be part of a PE programme such as dance and sport?
4. Is there a coherent study route through secondary to further and higher education for these PE related areas which involves all phases in the development and delivery of course content to avoid duplication of study.
5. Should GCSE PE be considered to be an optional extra to a school PE programme or, as a foundation subject in the National Curriculum, be available to all pupils in all secondary schools?

While the development of these courses has raised concerns, there are many positive aspects associated with those who are either planning, delivering, or receiving these courses.

They include: the opportunity of being involved in the issue of assessment in PE; the opportunity of widening the traditional school PE programme; introducing areas of learning which could lead pupils to advanced study and vocational opportunities; keeping PE teachers involved in mainstream developments in education (eg GCSE); and demonstrating to staff, pupils and parents the width of study in PE and its inter-disciplinary nature.

To conclude this section one feature which relates to all these courses should be considered. Concerns have often been expressed about the 'theoretical' or 'academic' content of these courses, in the sense that if a course is part of a physical education programme it should be about movement and activity and not about learning in a classroom. The issue, I would suggest, is presenting course content in an interesting and relevant manner which conveys the essence of the subject to the learner by promoting understanding and enthusiasm which instils a thirst for further knowledge and involvement. Therefore, it is much more relevant for young people to learn about, for example, acquisition of physical skills by a combination of practical experiments, discussion and reflection rather than just studying written information. The same could also be said for such areas of study as 'the effects of exercise on the body' or 'training and fitness' and many areas associated with 'contemporary issues' (ie politics, sponsorship, the media and spectator behaviour) could benefit from the teaching approach associated with B TEC courses which are assignment based and encourage active learning.

I would also suggest that it is wrong to assume specialist PE staff will automatically have the experience and knowledge to teach these courses effectively. There are important INSET implications to update or introduce knowledge and relate this to planning, delivery and pitch.

The other feature to be considered is the availability of appropriate resource materials. To date, the popularity of the few first level books written to resource GCSE-type courses in PE demonstrates the market need for this type of resource.

Finally, a debate has raged for many years as to whether physical education should associate with any form of examination work in schools. The major thrust of this argument revolves around the concern that examination courses would inhibit the physical experience, which is the major contribution PE makes to the whole educational process, by having to conform to the requirements of a prescribed syllabus and assessment procedures which may not be compatible with the subject! For example, written examination papers. While I would hope we would all share that concern, many would suggest that, when taught in an appropriate manner, examination courses can enrich a pupil's physical education. They can also enable the concepts of knowledge, understanding and skills associated with PE to be demonstrated to pupils in a relevant form to enhance their own perceptions of the interdisciplinary nature of this subject.

To conclude, I would suggest that if we agree that the content of a course represents areas of learning which are relevant and valid to the needs of students and society, then the public examination system is merely an administrative vehicle to demonstrate, in a nationally recognised way, the level of achievement and understanding of pupils who have undertaken that course of study. The issue is therefore not to allow the examination tail to wag the subject dog.

Records of achievement

By the end of 1991 it is the government's intention that a 'mechanism be in place' to enable all pupils leaving school at 16 to have a record of achievement which is a summative document, based on formative process, representing a complete 'record' of that person and their experiences. One such example of this has been developed by The West Midlands Examination Board (Midland Record of Achievement). A significant feature of this scheme is that schools may submit 'courses' to the board which can receive accreditation and be included in the final record of achievement.

The 14 to 16 Project (DES – LAPP) in Sandwell Education Authority, has produced a range of these courses which relate to physical education. These include units of work for several different sports and health related fitness.

Apart from the pupils receiving recognition of levels of achievement from the examination board, there are other significant features provided by this scheme.

As with some other curriculum initiatives MRA provides a framework for the submission to be written in. Each unit has to describe, under four headings, a series of outcomes to be addressed by each pupil. These headings are as follows:

1. Knowledge (the student has demonstrated knowledge of . . .).
2. Skills (the student has demonstrated the ability to . . .).
3. Concepts (the student has demonstrated an understanding of . . .).
4. Experiences (the student has experience of . . .).

The assessment procedures for these schemes can be decided by the course authors in consultation with the Board. An example from this scheme is provided by Appendix 9.1, which illustrates a unit stage from a Team Sports Scheme.

Planning courses in the context of this framework has provided teachers with the opportunity to consider activities which form part of a physical education programme, in a more critical way. This has resulted in courses which provide a wider range of learning opportunities than is normally associated with traditional senior school work.

It is this feature of the Midland Record of Achievement which leads to a curriculum model for the accreditation of all upper school areas of study (Figure 9.2). This provides units of work in all programme areas which is suitable for all levels of intellectual and physical ability, which should be the broad base for the whole programme.

These units can be made compatible with the content of GCSE courses so that pupils who have achieved at an appropriate level can be entered with the Examination Board for either section 2, MRA certification or GCSE physical education. Involvement in representative competition, sports clubs and sports events can also contribute to this document. The study route could then take pupils into either Advanced Level courses or vocational study during the 16 to 18 phase.

This model need only affect the Physical Education Department. However, if a whole school approach is adopted a variety of GCSE options can be provided within a limited time allocation.

For example, using the Midland Examination Board GCSE Theory and Practice of Physical Education course, it is possible to provide the following 'theory' units which could be compatible with the course but could contribute also to other courses.

1. Anatomy and physiology, the effect of exercise and treatment of injury could all contribute to science or human biology courses.

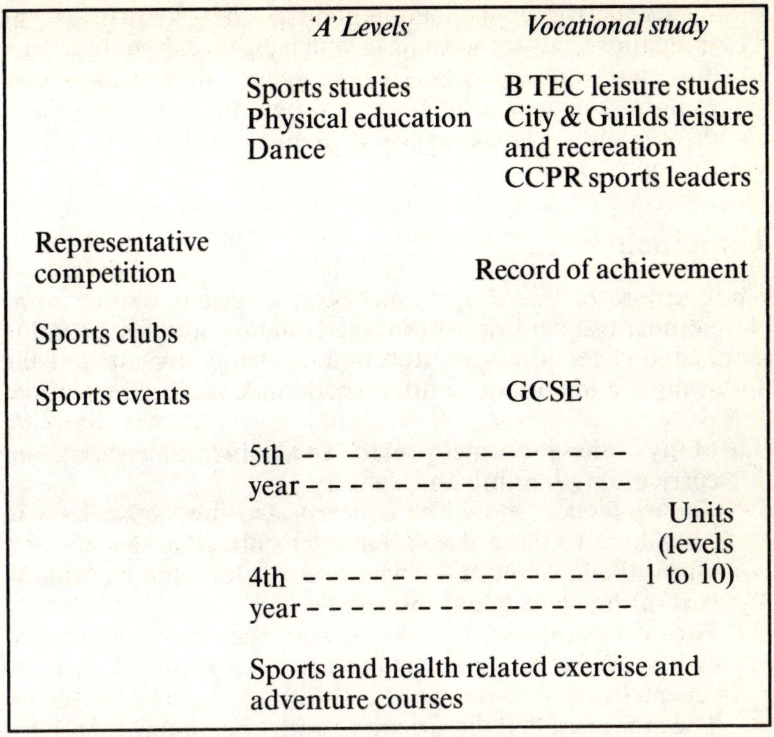

	'A' Levels	Vocational study
	Sports studies Physical education Dance	B TEC leisure studies City & Guilds leisure and recreation CCPR sports leaders
Representative competition		Record of achievement
Sports clubs		
Sports events		GCSE
	5th - - - - - - - - - - - - - - - year - - - - - - - - - - - - - - -	
		Units (levels
	4th - - - - - - - - - - - - - - year - - - - - - - - - - - - -	1 to 10)
	Sports and health related exercise and adventure courses	

Figure 9.2 *An accredited framework for Physical Education 14 to 18*

2. The role of sport in politics, sponsorship, the media and spectator behaviour could all contribute to social studies, media studies or sociology courses.
3. Acquisition of skill can feature as part of a psychology course.
4. Training and fitness and the effects of external influences on performance (eg drugs) could also feature in a health studies course.

The result could be a system where, if units were presented using individualised methods and with the different requirements of examination courses addressed, it would be possible to accommodate all 'theory' areas of the course, allowing the practical work to be covered during 'normal' PE time.

An alternative could be similar to that known as the Leicestershire Modular Scheme, in which pupils can study a series of short courses or modules (10 to 12 weeks), all accredited with an examination board, to form a programme with sufficient depth, breadth, coherence and quality to lead to GCSE certification.

Conclusions

The purpose of this chapter has been to briefly outline some development and ideas within accreditation and its planning implications for physical education. I would suggest that the following are important features which are concerned with this:

1. Many of these schemes provide a valuable framework to aid curriculum planning and delivery.
2. The profession should be concerned to investigate ways to contribute to these developments to illustrate the place of physical education in the whole curriculum and its value as part of the educational process.
3. The wide range of learning experiences in physical education can be enhanced by the structures provided by these schemes.
4. The argument that these courses and schemes provide status for the subject is irrelevant. What we should be promoting is that physical education enriches the range of these courses by taking its place with them.
5. To distance or isolate our subject from these developments will not be to the benefit of physical education, its teachers or its pupils. The issue is to develop courses which enable the 'nature' of the subject to be retained within a nationally or locally designed framework.

With the advent of a National Curriculum and the requirement to raise standards and provide evidence of achievement, the school curriculum will be subject to considerable attention and revue during the next few years. The physical education profession can provide a lead to other subject areas by demonstrating how structures for accreditation can be utilised to promote or support good practice. However, there will be a need for all of those associated with physical education to support and share with each other for the future development of our subject.

Appendix 9.1 is an example of a unit stage (level 3) of a series of three unit stages which form one unit.

Appendix 9.1
The West Midlands Examinations Board Record of Achievement

List of Unit Outcomes

Scheme title: SPORTS AND LEISURE

References		Number of units in scheme:

Unit reference	Unit title	Unit stage
S3	ASSOCIATION FOOTBALL	3

Knowledge

The student has demonstrated knowledge of:

1. The levels of organisation for any sport, eg Local Association, Regional Association, National Association and International Association.
2. The four elements that should be included in a training session, eg warm up, individual skill practices, conditioning, games sessions.
3. Two attacking skills and two defensive skills used when playing soccer, eg shooting, dribbling, marking and tackling.

4. The following terms:
   A 'Drill' as being a practice for a specified individual skill. 'Group work' as being any skill practice/activity requiring students to work together.
5. The two practices that can be used to improve a given basic skill, eg individual, partnerwork, small side games.
6. The various organisational factors involved in a skill practice for a small group, ie equipment, key coaching points.
7. Two tactics commonly used in soccer.
8. A playing system commonly used in soccer.

Skills

9. Describe a skill practice to improve a basic skill.
10. Demonstrate at least ONE ATTACKING and ONE DEFENSIVE SKILL.
11. Apply the major rules and scoring while refereeing a period of a practice game.
12. Find information about opportunities to be involved with soccer outside school.

Concepts

The student has demonstrated an understanding of:

13. A playing system – as being the way a team is organised positionally when playing a game.
14. Every sport having a governing body at either national or international level who is responsible for formulating the rules of the game.
15. How the National Association for a particular sport links up with each local association via regional associations.

Experiences

The student has experiences of:

16. General teaching about how to improve the level of basic skill and the major rules needed to play soccer.
17. Taking an active part in warm ups prior to playing the game.

18. Taking an active part in skill practices including taking some responsibility as a group leader or captain.
19. Using the equipment required to play soccer.
20. Taking an active part in a game.
21. Refereeing/umpiring and scoring for a period of a game.